SIMKIN

HANDBOOK OF THERAPEUTIC MONITORING

Second Edition

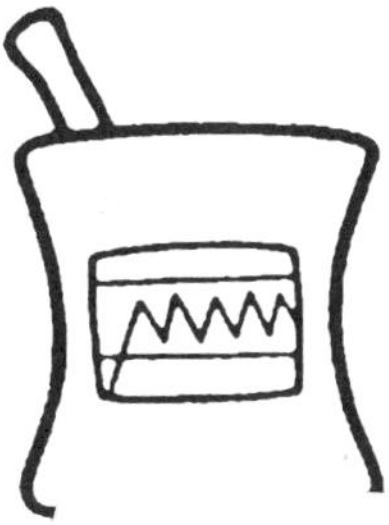

Edited by

William J. Taylor, Pharm.D.

J. Daniel Robinson, Pharm.D.

Susan Spivey-Miller

IMPORTANT: Note the Following Information Before Using This Handbook.

The purpose of this handbook is to assist the clinician in the interpretation of serum drug concentration data using professional judgment in view of available clinical information. Although the information contained in this handbook has been obtained from highly reputable sources and is believed to be accurate in accordance with currently available information, the publisher, the editors, and Simkin, Inc., assume no liability in connection with the use of any specific information contained herein. Complete information available from the drug manufacturers concerning indications, mechanism of action, methods of administration, dosages, modes and timing of elimination, and adverse effects of therapeutic drugs should be consulted.

Simkin, Inc.
408 W. University Ave., Suite 301
Gainesville, FL 32601

Second Edition.

Library of Congress Catalog Card Number: 93-83709
International Standard Book Number: 0-929375-10-6

EDITORS

William J. Taylor, Pharm.D.
Clinical Associate Professor of Neurology
University of South Alabama
Mobile, Alabama

J. Daniel Robinson, Pharm.D.
Professor of Pharmacy
College of Pharmacy
University of Florida
Gainesville, Florida

Susan Spivey-Miller
Pharm.D. Candidate
College of Pharmacy
University of Florida
Gainesville, Florida

TABLE OF CONTENTS

PREFACE

Seldom in modern medicine is routine and unvaried prescribing of an average dose of a pharmacologic agent completely satisfactory. Today it is well accepted that the therapeutic and toxic effects of a pharmacologic agent involve a multiplicity of objective and subjective variables. In a broad sense these variables include the pharmacokinetic properties of the drug, patient-specific parameters, and the disease process. An understanding of the basic pharmacokinetic concepts, such as biologic half-life, clearance, and bioavailability, is essential for one to effectively characterize the behavior of a drug within the body. A fundamental knowledge of an agent's pharmacodynamics and clearly defined therapeutic endpoints is equally essential for rational pharmacotherapeutics. Furthermore, patient-specific parameters and disease processes may alter the pharmacokinetics, the pharmacodynamics, and even the therapeutic endpoints. Therefore, a thorough knowledge of these interrelationships is necessary for optimal patient management. The clinical application of basic pharmacokinetics and pharmacodynamics allows the clinician to reduce the variability of drug behavior in an individual patient.

To clinically apply basic pharmacotherapeutic principles, the factors that alter the pharmacokinetics and pharmacodynamics of a specific pharmacological agent must be understood. The factors include a number of patient characteristics, a variety of clinically important drug interactions, and a few physical alterations in the drug product. Specific patient characteristics known to influence the effects of a drug are age, sex, pregnancy, genetics, and several disease processes. Clinically significant drug interactions occur principally through pharmacokinetic alterations and receptor site inhibition or potentiation. Physical alterations of a drug product play only a minor role in pharmacotherapeutics, but should be considered when an unexpected patient response is seen.

Once the principles of pharmacokinetics and pharmacodynamics are understood, the obvious objective is the individualization of dosages to maximize the efficacy and safety of drug therapy. Ideally, individualization of drug therapy is best accomplished by titration of dosage to the appropriate pharmacologic response. However, there are many inherent problems in attempting to quantify an adequate pharmacologic response. This difficulty may be overcome in many cases by the use of serum drug concentrations, pharmacokinetic software designed by Simkin, Inc. and good clinical judgment.

The basic intent of this handbook is to acquaint the reader with the pharmacokinetic parameters that are used in the development of rational therapeutic drug monitoring. In order to accomplish this goal, we begin this handbook with a discussion of the major components of pharmacokinetics and pharmacodynamics that influence each drug's behavior in the body. Following that discussion are sets of tables on a variety of drugs that require individualized dosing. All numerical values for pharmacokinetic parameters are approximations derived from various sources. They should be used for beginning estimates and revised once serum drug concentrations are obtained on an individual patient.

LIST OF ABBREVIATIONS

Following is a list of commonly used pharmacokinetic and medical abbreviations which may be used throughout this and similar texts:

A	Amount of drug in the body
A_u	Amount of drug in the urine
AF	Atrial fibrillation
AUC	Area under the curve from time zero to infinity following a single dose
BP	Blood pressure
BUN	Blood urea nitrogen
C	Concentration
$C_{avg,ss}$	Average steady-state concentration
C_{max}	Concentration maximum (peak)
C_{min}	Concentration minimum (trough)
$C_{max,ss}$	Maximum (peak) steady-state concentration
$C_{min,ss}$	Minimum (trough) steady-state concentration
C_{ss}	Steady-state concentration
C_{ther}	Therapeutic range concentration
C_{tox}	Toxic concentration (generally lowest)
$C_{u,ss}$	Average steady-state concentration of unbound drug
CBC	Complete blood count
CHF	Congestive heart failure
Cl	Clearance
CL_{cr}	Creatinine clearance
Cl_{int}	Hepatic intrinsic clearance
Cl_h	Hepatic clearance
Cl_r	Renal clearance

CNS	Central nervous system
D	Dose
D/τ	Dose rate
E	Hepatic extraction ratio
ECG	Electrocardiogram
f	Bioavailable fraction
f_u	Unbound drug fraction in serum, plasma, or blood
f_{ut}	Unbound drug fraction in "tissue"
GFR	Glomerular filtration rate
GI	Gastrointestinal
Ig	Immunoglobulin (e.g. IgA, IgG, IgM)
IM	Intramuscular
IV	Intravenous route of administration
K	Elimination rate constant
kg	kilogram
K_o	Rate of constant (zero-order) infusion
K_m	Michaelis constant
L	Liter
μg	Microgram
mEq	Milliequivalent
mg	Milligram
mL	Milliliter
NAPA	N-acetyl procainamide
ng	Nanogram
nl	Normal
PO	Oral route of administration

prn	As needed
PVC	Premature ventricular contractions
Q	Hepatic blood flow
τ	Dosing interval
RBC	Red blood cell count
S_{cr}	Serum creatinine
SDC	Serum drug concentrations
SLE	Systemic lupus erythematosus
t	Time
t'	Time at end of infusion
$t_{1/2}$	Elimination half-life
$t_{50\%}$	Time to eliminate 50% of drug from the body (nonlinear elimination)
TSH	Thyroid-stimulating hormone
V_c	Central volume of distribution
V_d	Apparent volume of distribution
V_{ss}	Steady-state volume of distribution
V_t	Tissue volume
V_{max}	Maximum rate of metabolism
WBC	White blood cell count

GENERAL PRINCIPLES AND CONCEPTS

GENERAL PRINCIPLES AND CONCEPTS

One of the most important aspects of drug action in the body is termed "pharmacokinetics." An understanding of this process enables clinicians to design and adjust drug doses for their patients. It also helps clinicians anticipate and resolve problems of drug toxicity or interactions. According to the traditional definition, pharmacokinetics is the quantitative study of the metabolic process of drug absorption, distribution, biotransformation, and elimination. The use of mathematical models to describe these processes allows predictions about drug concentrations in various parts of the body as a function of dosage, route of administration, and time.

When clinically applied, pharmacokinetics (*clinical pharmacokinetics*) is an effective aid to clinicians in achieving optimal treatment with selected therapeutic agents. A serum drug concentration (SDC) determination collected at the proper time and interpreted in the proper pharmacokinetic and clinical context is a major step toward individualizing dosages for many drugs.

Many factors must be considered when interpreting SDC, since each patient has specific characteristics (e.g., genotype, coexisting disease, concomitant drug therapy) that may affect SDC. The relationship between drug dosage and resulting concentrations in serum will also be influenced by such factors as the bioavailability of the dosage form used, patient body size, distribution through fluid compartments, and individual metabolic and excretion rates.

There are a number of key concepts that the reader should understand in order to effectively use this handbook in conjunction with a computerized pharmacokinetic system and manual.

INITIATION OF A THERAPEUTIC DRUG MONITORING (TDM) SERVICE

There are several possible criteria for referring patients to a TDM service. The first and most desirable method is by physician consultation. The advantage of this method is that the program and advice provided is desired by the requesting physician. Thus, there is obviously greater acceptability of the recommendations. Another important advantage is that reimbursement from insurance companies often requires the consult to be initiated by a physician.

A large percentage of services and/or referrals are initiated through specific monitoring programs. The program may be specialized; for example, it may include only patients receiving aminoglycoside antibiotics or patients who have had their theophylline concentrations determined. Evaluation of and recommendations for concentrations that fall outside a specific range is another reason for initiating a TDM service. An ideal approach would be for pharmacists to use a computer system that checks the prescription order against the patient's database to determine if the current dosage regimen is predictive of abnormal SDC.

Which drugs should be monitored? Those that can be accurately and readily measured, and meet the criteria below. Some of these include:

Amikacin	*Carbamazepine*	*Digoxin*
Gentamicin/Tobramycin	*Lidocaine*	*Lithium*
Phenobarbital/Primidone	*Phenytoin*	*Theophylline*
Procainamide/NAPA	*Quinidine*	*Vancomycin*
Valproic Acid		

Information on most of the above drugs currently is available in your pharmacokinetic system. These agents can be divided into *two groups.* The *first* of the therapeutic agent groups includes agents that exhibit an erratic and/or unpredictable dose-response relationship; for example, individual variations in phenytoin metabolic rates create marked variability in SDC in patients with similar demographic profiles and similar seizure disorders, even though all patients are dosed with the same milligram/kilogram dose. Phenytoin is a good example of a therapeutic agent whose efficacy is at times difficult to evaluate, especially since seizure occurrence can be paroxysmal. The *second* group of therapeutic agents includes those that possess a narrow therapeutic-toxic range. A classic example are the aminoglycosides. Individualized dosing is necessary not only to ensure the probability of efficacy but also to help prevent serious toxicity.

Clinical application of therapeutic drug monitoring is limited to agents demonstrating a correlation between a particular range of SDC and a beneficial therapeutic effect. There are several *indications* that are useful in determining whether SDC should be monitored:

- When drug efficacy is questioned
- When a patient exhibits possible drug-related toxicity
- When noncompliance is suspected
- When a patient has a concomitant disease that may alter drug disposition
- When a drug-drug interaction is suspected
- When establishing a baseline value after a patient exhibits a satisfactory response to drug therapy
- When changing dosage formulation or adjusting a dosage regimen
- When a patient's condition is refractory to a dosage regimen

In addition to designing criteria for initiating a defined TDM service, some clinicians have attempted to screen samples prior to analysis in order to decrease the number of assays run for inappropriate reasons.

Inappropriate testing has been a major problem not only in drug assays, but in laboratory tests in general. Therefore, TDM services develop specific criteria that must be adhered to before a sample will be analyzed. General criteria for obtaining a sample for drug analysis include (1) an evaluation of the appropriateness of an administered loading or maintenance dose; (2) an evaluation of a suboptimal drug response; and (3) an evaluation of a potential drug-induced toxicity.

DRUG HALF-LIFE (T 1/2)

The half-life of a drug is the time required for the drug's peak SDC to decline by 50%. A drug's half-life is used in determining when to collect SDC samples from patients and in designing dosing regimens.

STEADY-STATE LEVELS (C_{ss})

Steady-state levels are important in chronic drug therapy. When repeated doses of a drug are given at regular intervals, serum levels will rise until equilibrium is reached between the dose administered and the amount eliminated. This level is the steady-state SDC and is usually achieved after three to five half-lives of a given drug. The times to steady-state given in this volume (e.g., five times the average elimination half-life) are averages, and they can be affected by various disease states and co-administered agents that alter the drug's half-life.

THERAPEUTIC RANGE (C_{ther})

Therapeutic ranges for a number of drugs have been established. For each of these drugs, clinical correlation has demonstrated a minimum SDC below which the desired drug effect is usually not seen, and a maximum SDC above which toxic effects are likely to outweigh therapeutic benefit. Due to individual variations in drug disposition, some patients tolerate—and may require—serum levels above or below a drug's therapeutic range to achieve the desired therapeutic effect.

PEAK AND TROUGH CONCENTRATIONS (C_{max}, C_{min})

Most dosage regimens will produce a peak/trough pattern in SDC. A "*peak*" sample theoretically represents the maximum drug concentration during a dosing interval, while a "*trough*" sample theoretically represents the lowest level. The peak concentration usually is measured after the drug distribution phase is completed to assure that the concentration is within the therapeutic range, not above or below it. The trough concentration usually is measured just prior to the next dose to ensure that the SDC is above the minimum effective concentration or that the drug is being eliminated from the body at an appropriate rate (e.g., aminoglycosides).

- With drugs whose SDC levels are described as peaks and troughs (e.g., aminoglycosides), the doses are often administered every 8h. It is better to obtain both values during the same dosing interval because there are fewer variables. However, waiting 8h to take the trough sample delays the results, usually causes the results to be affected by variance in laboratory personnel, and is more time consuming for the phlebotomist. The practical aspects of obtaining SDC levels often conflict with pharmacokinetic theory. Consequently, most institutions obtain aminoglycoside SDC levels by drawing the trough sample 30 min prior to a dose, and the peak 30 min after the end of the IV bolus infusion.

Exact times corresponding to the highest and lowest drug concentrations within a dosing interval vary from patient to patient, and with different preparations of the same drug. Therefore, all sampling times cited in this handbook are estimates. Peak and trough concentrations can be calculated exactly by utilizing your computerized pharmacokinetic system.

SAMPLING CONSIDERATIONS

Timing of Sampling

The timing of blood sampling in relation to dosage is critical for correct interpretation of the SDC result. Collection time should be based on the pharmacokinetic properties of the drug, its dosage form (e.g., intravenous solution, intramuscular injection, oral tablet), the dosing protocol, and the clinical reason for assaying the sample. Improper sampling can often lead to incorrect interpretation and erroneous therapeutic adjustments. For example, a high therapeutic value prior to a gentamicin IV dose would be interpreted differently from the same value drawn after the dose. Low values obtained prior to steady-state may cause the clinician to dangerously increase the dose. Drugs with long half-lives require different sampling techniques than those with short half-lives. Misinterpretation also can be attributed to sampling performed during the distribution and/or absorption phase. Peak concentration levels depend upon timing and route of administration. For example, peak SDC following an IV dose of theophylline may occur within minutes after injection, whereas it may not occur for 6–8h for a sustained-release product such as Theo-Dur. The patient should be at steady-state (3–5 elimination half-lives) when a sample is collected to ensure reliable interpretation of SDC.

Timing of peak SDC levels is dependent on the drug product. IV bolus injections peak rapidly. Therefore, a true peak SDC can be obtained in the opposite arm from administration once blood circulation time is complete—within a few minutes for drugs with single-compartment kinetics (e.g. phenobarbital and heparin). However, *most drugs obey two-compartment kinetics,* and therapeutic effect usually correlates with SDC levels obtained after the alpha (distribution) phase. Therefore, when peaks are defined within clinical context, they generally are obtained 20 to 30 min (30 to 60 min for aminoglycosides) after IV injection even though they are not the true pharmacokinetic peaks. The period for aminoglycosides is longer because they are normally intravenously infused over 30 min. This 30-min period is followed by a distribution phase that is approximately 30 min. Consequently, peak aminoglycoside SDC levels are usually obtained 30 or 60 min after the completion of infusion.

Peak concentrations of dosage forms other than IV bolus injections must include consideration of absorption and distribution phases. Intramuscular injections usually peak within 30–60 min. However, some intramuscular injections peak unpredictably with variable bioavailable quantities (i.e., they are absorbed more slowly than oral dosage). For this reason, intramuscular injections of digoxin should be avoided. Liquid oral dosages, e.g., digoxin elixir and theophylline elixir, are usually absorbed very quickly and liquid dosages may peak within a 30-min period. Peak theophylline levels after oral solid doses can occur at 30–60 min, whereas the digoxin clinical peak (post-distribution) occurs 6h after a tablet. This occurs because distribution of theophylline is much faster than digoxin. Solid oral dosage forms may be available in rapid- and slow-release varieties. Rapid absorption forms such as quinidine sulfate peak at approximately one to 2h after dosage. However, slow-release forms peak in 3–4h. Concomitant food ingestion or drugs can delay the peak of many products 30–60 min.

Timing of trough SDC levels also depends on the drug product. Trough concentrations are clinically defined as SDC that is obtained prior to the next dose. True trough concentration may actually occur within the next dosage interval, because the SDC continues to fall while the next dose is dissolving and being absorbed *(lag time).* This fact is generally ignored in the clinical setting. IV bolus injections do not have lag time and the SDC obtained prior to the next dose is the true trough. It is difficult for the laboratory to time the sample collection immediately prior to the administration of the drug. Practical considerations may cause a significant difference between true trough and measured trough in drugs with short half-lives. Aminoglycosides have an average half-life of 2h, for example, which causes the SDC to fall 10% to 15% in 30 min (50% x 0.5 hr/2 hr). Consequently, a trough obtained 30 min early may be measured as 2.1 μg/mL (toxic) while the true trough actually is 1.9 μg/mL (which may be interpreted as therapeutic).

Other Factors Affecting Sampling

There are several other factors that influence sample collection:

- Certain commercial *blood collection tubes* may affect drug concentration in whole blood samples. It has been suggested that a plasticizer leaches from their stoppers into the whole blood sample where it displaces the drug from its plasma-binding sites, causing a redistribution of the drug into erythrocytes. Subsequent measurement of the sample's plasma drug level may result in an artificially lowered concentration. Use all-glass tubes or test any commercial collection tube thoroughly before utilization.

- Use of heparinized tubes to collect specimens for aminoglycoside analysis is controversial. Until the controversy is resolved, *the use of non-heparinized tubes is recommended.*

- When a specimen is collected during an infusion, the sample should be taken from the opposite limb.

TDM MONITORING FORM

The TDM monitoring form is a key tool for the interpretation of therapeutic drug monitoring data. It must be well designed to encourage the entry of important clinical information as well as providing space for SDC measurements and ranges. The form should contain a variety of drug information, such as:

Specific Patient Information
- Name and address
- Identification numbers
- Physician and specialty

Patient Characteristics
- Age, sex, pregnancy, ethnicity
- Height and weight
- Allergies
- Primary disease process
- Organ involvement, especially renal, hepatobiliary, gastrointestinal, cardiac, or endocrine
- Fluid balance
- Laboratory studies, creatinine clearance and serum albumin, etc.

Specimen Information

- Time of collection
- Nature of specimen: blood, urine, other body fluids
- Site of collection
- Order of sample, if one of a series
- Type of container, preservative

Drug Information

- Name of drug(s) to be assayed
- Time of last dose, frequency of prescribed dose, quantity of dose, route of administration
- Concomitant drug therapy

Purpose of Assay and Urgency of Request

- Therapeutic confirmation
- Suspected toxicity
- Drug overdose
- Monitoring active metabolites
- Suspected drug interactions
- Comprehensive pharmacokinetic evaluation and consultation
- Absence of therapeutic response, which may be due to drug failure, noncompliance, altered clearance, or altered absorption

INTERPRETATION AND CONSULTATION

Substantial data exist that indicate clinicians frequently may not use assay results appropriately when making dosage decisions. *Most errors occur when a dosage change is made based upon a sample that was drawn improperly.* In addition, clinicians sometimes fail to make incremental dosage increases accordingly when subtherapeutic levels are reported. Rather than maximizing the therapeutic benefits of one drug, they often add a second drug. Because of these factors, active participation by the clinician in interpreting drug assay results is encouraged. An absolute minimal level of service would be reporting the toxic drug concentrations directly to the primary care physician as quickly as possible. In clinical usage, therapeutic drug monitoring is somewhat analogous to the ECG or radiograph, where the interpretation of the test is as important as the procedure itself. The clinician should treat the patient, not the SDC. A value outside the therapeutic range should provoke a reassessment. To fully utilize an assay, results must be interpreted in light of the complete clinical situation, using all available information. *The following is a list of factors that can affect SDC interpretation:*

- Dosage regimen and dosage form of each drug
- Patient age, weight, and sex
- Time the sample was obtained
- Time elapsed since last administration of drug being measured
- Whether the SDC represents a steady-state concentration
- Whether the level represents free or total drug concentration (using available techniques, SDC are reported as total concentrations, i.e., free plus protein-bound drug)
- Whether the SDC is a peak or trough concentration
- Route of administration
- Individual drug pharmacokinetic parameters
- Multiple disease processes
- Concomitant drug therapy
- Alcohol intake
- Clinical status of the patient

Most of the data manipulation and use of complex equations required to provide adequate service can be performed on microcomputers. Appropriate software can quickly solve cumbersome equations that can be used either for parameter estimation or data simulation, and the computer can print hard-copy consult records and store patient information for subsequent retrieval or data analysis for research purposes.

After appropriate interpretation of results, decisions concerning patient therapy need to be communicated effectively to the physician provider. The specific degree of involvement depends on legal requirements, hospital policy, and political considerations. Most services operate either as consulting or monitoring services. The ultimate decision, however, rests with the attending physician. *The degree of success, therefore, depends primarily on the development of a strong collaborative working relationship with physicians in each institution.*

Recommendations optimally are discussed with the attending physician. This will assure full understanding of the situation and will allow the physician to have questions answered. This interaction also provides an opportunity to obtain further insight into the patient's clinical condition and identify the specific therapeutic goals of the physician. The information gained can often change the approach to a given patient. This type of communication should always be cooperative, not condescending, and should provide a strong basis for a good working relationship between physicians and those involved in TDM. Whenever specific verbal recommendations are made, written documentation of the interaction should be placed in the patient chart.

There are basically two levels of consultation. The most fundamental level involves *minimal interpretation* of the SDC. The questions answered by this type of consult usually include:

- Appropriateness of sample time
- The usual therapeutic range
- Factors that influence the total concentration
- Unbound concentration (i.e., protein binding)
- The expected level, based on pharmacokinetic parameters
- Accuracy of assay results

This type of interpretation is essential for all SDC consultations and should not be minimized. A more *in-depth consult* is needed for many patients, to develop recommendations regarding the design of individualized dosing regimens. This includes dosing history, SDC information, the patient's status (including objective and subjective signs), therapeutic or lack of therapeutic effect, drug toxicity, and a pharmacokinetic analysis. Specific recommendations are:

- Dosage adjustment
- Follow-up SDC data
- Specific laboratory or other monitoring parameters

Recommendations should not be made solely on the basis of the SDC.

Other concepts necessary to understand and use TDM optimally are listed in the glossary.

AMIKACIN

CLINICAL PHARMACOKINETICS

SUMMARY TABLE

SERUM CONCENTRATIONS		
Moderate-severe systemic infection (Minimum effective concentrations)	Peak concentration Trough concentration	20–25 μg/mL 1–4 μg/mL
Life-threatening systemic infection (Minimum effective concentrations)	Peak concentration Trough concentration	25–30 μg/mL 5–8 μg/mL
Potentially toxic concentrations	Peak concentrations Trough concentration	> 30 μg/mL > 8 μg/mL
TIME TO PEAK CONCENTRATION	IM administration IV administration	0.5–1 h Immediately post-infusion
TIME TO STEADY-STATE	Variable	Generally achieved in 4–5 half-lives
HALF-LIFE (T½)		
Normal renal function	Average S_{cr}≤1.5 mg/dL CL_{cr}≥100 mL/min/1.73m^2	2 h 0.5–15 h 0.5–8 h
Age	Neonates Children Adults ≤ 30 yr old Adults > 30 yr old	2–9 h 0.5–3 h 0.5–3 h 1.5–15 h
All ranges of renal function		0.7–70 h
VOLUME OF DISTRIBUTION		
Adults	Dehydration Normal fluid status Increased extracellular fluid	0.05–0.15 L/kg 0.15–0.25 L/kg 0.25–0.70 L/kg
Children Neonates		0.07–0.70 L/kg 0.20–0.70 L/kg
CLEARANCE		
Total body clearance	Normal S_{cr}(≤1.5 mg/dL) Abnormal S_{cr}(≥1.5 mg/dL) CL_{cr}≥100 mL/min	1.33 ± 0.61 mL/min/kg 0.53 ± 0.35 mL/min/kg 1.51 ± 0.60 mL/min/kg
Dialysis clearance	Hemodialysis 6h hemodialysis Peritoneal dialysis	30–60 mL/min 40–60% Less effective in removing aminoglycosides
% SERUM PROTEIN-BOUND		0–30%
% EXCRETED RENALLY UNCHANGED	Unchanged	85–95% (glomerular)

MAJOR ROUTE OF ELIMINATION AND ACTIVE METABOLITES	No known metabolites	Glomerular filtration, 85–95% of dose renally excreted as unchanged drug
HEPATIC METABOLISM	Percent of dose Active metabolites Toxic metabolites	Negligible None None

THERAPEUTIC DRUG MONITORING

GENERAL GUIDELINES

- The interpatient variability of amikacin pharmacokinetics, the seriousness of gram-negative infections, and the risk of toxicity require that patients be monitored closely. Both peak and trough concentrations should be monitored closely and dosages adjusted to attain desired SDC.

- A method exists that allows the clinician to calculate the dose and dosing interval from the SDC-time data, although the frequency of monitoring should be determined for each patient. Monitoring is indicated.

- Assess the adequacy of therapy based on therapeutic guidelines for a specific pathogen, site of infection, and clinical condition of the patient.

- To prevent excessively high SDC and reduce the risk of toxicity

- Renal function changes

- Changes in volume of distribution

- Dosage and/or dosing interval changes

SAMPLE COLLECTION

Peak	IM	60 min after injection
	IV	30 min after infusion or immediately after a 60-min infusion
Trough	IV	Immediately before administration of subsequent dose (under steady-state condition)

NOTE: SDCs may also reflect the patient's hydration status and changing renal function.

CLINICAL COMMENTS

- Both peak and trough concentrations should be measured over the same dosing interval.
- Sampling is often done prior to attainment of steady-state to help prevent toxicity and to ensure therapeutic efficacy.
- The use of heparinized tubes to collect specimens for aminoglycosides analysis is controversial. Until the controversy is resolved, heparinized tubes should not be used to collect specimens.
- High concentrations of beta-lactam antibiotics (penicillins) inactivate aminoglycosides in vivo and in vitro. Specimens containing a beta-lactam antibiotic in addition to an aminoglycoside should be either assayed immediately using a rapid method or stored frozen.

CLINICAL MONITORING PARAMETERS

- Blood urea nitrogen (BUN)
- Serum creatinine (S_{cr})
- Maximum body temperature per 24-h period
- Hemoglobin/hematocrit
- X-rays
- Cultures and sensitivities
- Patient weight
- Fluid intake and output (I/O)
- White blood cell count (WBC) with differential
- Concomitant antibiotics and other potentially ototoxic or nephrotoxic drugs

THERAPEUTICS

USUAL DOSING PARAMETERS

PATIENT GROUP	INITIAL DOSE	DAILY MAINTENANCE	APPROXIMATE T½ NORMAL RENAL FUNCTION
Pediatric		10–15 mg/kg/d	0.7–3.0 h
Dehydrated	5–7.5 mg/kg		
Normal hydration	7.5 mg/kg		
Increased extracellular fluid	7.5–10 mg/kg		
Normal renal function		10–15 mg/kg/d	0.7–3.0 h
Abnormal renal function		variable	variable
Neonates	10–18 mg/kg	12 mg/kg/d	variable
Adult 1.0–7.0 h		5–35 mg/kg/d	
Dehydrated	5–7.5 mg/kg		
Normal hydration	7.5 mg/kg		
Increased extracellular fluid	7.5–10 mg/kg		
Normal renal 1.0–7.0 h function		5–35 mg/kg/d	
Abnormal renal function		Adjust according to renal function	variable

CLINICAL COMMENTS

- These are suggested starting dosages. They may exceed manufacturer's recommendations and reflect opinions of usual dosages required to achieve therapeutic SDC in patients with serious infections and normal renal function. The monitoring of SDC is required. In neonates the dosage is based on gestational age and body weight.

- Dosing intervals should be adjusted based on patient response, SDC, and renal function.

- Administer in 2 or 3 divided doses. In patients with abnormal renal function, adjust dosage according to renal status and SDC.

- If administered intravenously, infuse over 30–60 min.

- Usual therapeutic range will be dependent on infecting organism, site of infection, immunological status of the patient, and severity of infection.

- Dosage requirements will vary depending on birth-weight and maturity; SDC should be monitored.

- With abnormal renal function, half-life is quite variable.

COMMON TOXICITIES AND ADVERSE REACTIONS

TOXICITY	RISK FACTORS	CLINICAL COMMENTS
Ototoxicity (Incidence: 1–2%)	Concomitant ototoxic drugs Prior exposure to aminoglycosides Duration of treatment > 10–18 days Cumulative dose > 15–25 g Average daily dose > 25 mg/kg Frequent peak plasma concentrations > 32 µg/mL Frequent trough plasma concentrations > 10 µg/mL Age > 60 years Renal insufficiency Dialysis	Ototoxicity is primarily cochlear but vestibular dysfunction also occurs. Most studies demonstrated the incidence of decreased hearing to be 2–10% by audiometry. Overt clinical toxicity is only about 1–2%. Auditory dysfunction is usually in the higher frequencies, but conversational hearing loss can occur. It is usually bilateral and permanent. Vestibular dysfunction usually manifests as slight vertigo or tinnitus, although acute Meniere's syndrome can occur. It is usually permanent. However, patients can overcome the dysfunction by compensatory mechanisms. They have greater difficulty ambulating in the dark.
Nephrotoxicity (Incidence: 3–10%)	Concomitant nephrotoxic drugs Prior exposure to aminoglycosides Total dose received > 15–25 g	Most studies demonstrated toxicity by an increase in serum creatinine and BUN. Overt nonoliguric renal failure occurs

TOXICITY	RISK FACTORS	CLINICAL COMMENTS
	Mean peak plasma concentrations > 16–20 μg/mL Highest peak plasma concentrations (20–40 μg/mL) Mean trough plasma concentration > 10 μg/mL Volume depletion Age > 60 years Renal insufficiency	infrequently, provided drug accumulation does not occur. Typical findings include a decreased glomerular filtration rate and impaired urinary concentrating ability. This usually occurs at least five days after initiating therapy. A Fanconi-like syndrome may occur.
Neuromuscular blockade (Incidence: Infrequent)	Concomitant administration of neuromuscular blocking agents and anesthetics In-patients with hypocalcemia Myasthenia gravis High SDC in newborns When administered intraperitoneally or rapid IV injection	Blockade is usually competitive, although a noncompetitive block may occur. Respiratory depression and apnea may be quickly reversed by administering calcium or anticholinesterase.
Other Adverse Effects		
Headache and Nausea (Incidence: < 1%)	Unknown	Reported reaction but of questionable association.
Abnormal liver function tests (Incidence: Rare)	Unknown	This reaction has been reported but is not definitely associated with therapy.

TOXICITY	RISK FACTORS	CLINICAL COMMENTS
Teratogenicity (Incidence: Infrequent)	Unknown	Not systematically studied...potential for ototoxicity and nephrotoxicity.
Tachycardia (Incidence: Infrequent)	Unknown	Questionable.
Allergic or Hypersensitivity Reactions (Incidence: 1–3%)	Possibly the length of the therapy	Rash, eosinophilia, and drug fever have been reported with incidence varying from 0.1% to 11%. However, the overall incidence may vary with the type of observation.

DRUG INTERACTIONS

DRUG	MECHANISM	CLINICAL COMMENTS
Amphotericin B	Synergistic nephrotoxicity may be exhibited	Patients receiving both agents concurrently should be closely monitored for renal function deterioration
Cephalosporins	Synergistic nephrotoxicity may be exhibited	May occur primarily with cephaloridine and cephalothin; closely monitor patient's renal function
Clindamycin	Likelihood of aminoglycoside nephrotoxicity which may be enhanced	Monitor patient's renal function carefully
Dimenhydrinate	Aminoglycoside ototoxicity may be masked	Monitor patient's cochlear and vestibular function carefully
Ethacrynic acid/furosemide	Aminoglycoside ototoxicity and nephrotoxicity may be potentiated	Monitor patient for ototoxicity and nephrotoxicity carefully
Heparin (>5–10 units/mL)	Chemical complex formation, usually reversible	Aminoglycoside concentration determinations may be erroneously low
Methoxyflurane	May include additive or synergistic nephrotoxicity	Monitor patient's renal function closely
Semisynthetic penicillins (carbenicillin, ticarcillin, piperacillin) and other beta-lactam antibiotics	Chemical complex formation, reversible	Aminoglycoside concentration determinations may be falsely low; may result in microbiologically inactive compounds; greatest effect may be seen with gentamicin and carbenicillin
Neuromuscular blocking agents and skeletal muscle relaxants	Aminoglycoside-induced neuromuscular blockade may be synergistic	Concurrent administration should be avoided since neuromuscular blockade may be enhanced; anticholinesterase agents may reverse the blockade

OTHER

A number of other agents may interact with amikacin, including vancomycin, polymyxins, furosemide, cisplatin, and general anesthesia

CLINICAL INTERPRETATION

Amikacin SDC data should be interpreted in the context of the patient's current clinical status, response, and other pharmacotherapeutic considerations. There are a number of factors that potentially alter the pharmacokinetics, therapeutics, and SDC of amikacin. These factors must be taken into consideration when determining monitoring frequency and the clinical interpretation of an amikacin SDC. They include:

MAY REQUIRE AN INCREASE IN DAILY DOSE

- Extremely burned patients
- Markedly obese individuals
- Patients with cystic fibrosis
- Patients with ascites
- Concomitant drug therapy; enzyme-inducing drugs, e.g., phenytoin (enhanced metabolism)
- Congestive heart failure
- Age (neonates have large apparent volume of distribution)
- Concomitant drug therapy: heparin (in vivo inactivation unlikely); high concentrations of certain penicillins, (e.g., carbenicillin, ticarcillin, and possibly ampicillin)----in vivo inactivation significant only in patients with renal failure

MAY REQUIRE A DECREASE IN DAILY DOSE

- Premature or underweight newborns
- Patients with reduced renal function
- Elderly patients
- Conditions associated with decreased volume of distribution (dehydration, etc.)

OTHER CONSIDERATIONS

- Recent myocardial infarction: initial SDC may be reduced (increased volume of distribution and prolonged elimination half-life)
- Collection tubes (see note in introduction)
- Peritonitis

CARBAMAZEPINE
(CBZ)

CLINICAL PHARMACOKINETICS

SUMMARY TABLE

SERUM CONCENTRATIONS		
Minimum effective concentration	**Note:** patients receiving multiple antiepileptics usually require concentrations between 4–8 μg/mL	4 μg/mL
Potentially toxic concentration		>8–12 μg/mL
% BIOAVAILABILITY		85–90%
TIME TO PEAK CONCENTRATION	A wide variability may exist between patients	3 h (1–15 h)
TIME TO STEADY-STATE*	After initiation of treatment	2–4 wk
	After dose/rate change	4–5 d
HALF-LIFE (T½)*	Monotherapy	12 h
	Combination therapy	4–5 h
VOLUME OF DISTRIBUTION		0.8–1.9 L/kg
CLEARANCE		
Total body clearance		
Adults		
Initial dose		11–26 mL/h/kg
Chronic therapy		50–100 mL/h/kg
Pediatrics		
Chronic therapy		50–400 mL/h/kg
Dialysis clearance	% removed during 6–hr hemodialysis	<2%
% PROTEIN-BOUND		67–81%
% EXCRETED RENALLY UNCHANGED		<1% excreted unchanged
MAJOR ROUTE OF ELIMINATION	Hepatic	99%
ACTIVE METABOLITES	Carbamazepine 10,11-epoxide, which has been shown to have antiepileptic activity in animals	25–50%

* Affected by the drug's known metabolic enzyme autoinduction properties.

THERAPEUTIC DRUG MONITORING

GENERAL GUIDELINES

If only one measurement is to be made, then the lowest plasma carbamazepine concentration during the dosage interval provides the best guide for dosage adjustment. Theoretically, this is represented by a trough level; however, due to the variability in carbamazepine absorption, the true trough may occur into the next oral dose.

Peak ~3h(patients on chronic oral therapy). Trough immediately before next dose.

	SERUM COLLECTION	CLINICAL COMMENTS
Initial Monitoring	2–4 wk after initiation	CBZ measured approximately 3 wk after initiation of therapy so that auto-induction is maximal and a true steady-state has been reached
Resampling Following dose/ rate changes	Before maximal auto-induction, 3–5 d After maximal auto-induction, 1–3 wk	Even if patient is responding to a new dose rate, important to establish the average concentration; provides reference point for future dosing rate adjustments
Following addition/ discontinuation of enzyme-inducer	1–2 wk later	A new steady-state will be reached in 1 to 2 wk
Evidence of toxicity or overdose	Immediately	Toxic concentration may be the only way to detect intoxication in a mentally retarded, comatose, or very young patient

	SERUM COLLECTION	CLINICAL COMMENTS
Loss of seizure control	Immediately, especially if overdose and paradoxical seizures are suspected	Concentration monitoring will also distinguish between inadequate antiepileptic therapy and seizures due to carbamazepine toxicity
Pregnancy	Frequently during and after delivery	Frequent plasma concentration monitoring provides a guide to rising dosing needs as a result of the progressive increase in carbamazepine body clearance during pregnancy; frequent monitoring 2 wk to 1 mo after delivery

CLINICAL MONITORING PARAMETERS

PARAMETER	CLINICAL COMMENTS
CBC with iron BUN and S_{cr}	Prior to initiation of therapy, weekly during the first 3 months of treatment, and periodically thereafter
Liver function tests Complete urinalysis	Prior to initiation of therapy and at periodic intervals during therapy
Ophthalmologic examination	Including slit-lamp, funduscopy, and tonometry prior to initiation and at periodic intervals during therapy

THERAPEUTICS

USUAL DOSING PARAMETERS

PATIENT GROUP	INITIAL DOSE	DAILY MAINTENANCE	APPROXIMATE T½ NORMAL RENAL FUNCTION
Pediatric (Children <15y of Age)			
Week 1	1/4–1/3 maintenance dose rate	11–40 mg/kg/d	5–27 h
Week 2	1/2–2/3 maintenance dose rate		
Week 3	3/4–all maintenance dose rate		
Adult			
Week 1	1/4–1/3 maintenance dose rate	7–15 mg/kg/d	5–27 h
Week 2	1/2–2/3 maintenance dose rate		
Week 3	3/4–all maintenance dose rate		

CLINICAL COMMENTS

♦ Initiation of Therapy, All Patients

No loading dose is advised. Dose rates should be gradually increased over 2–4 weeks according to one of the following schedules shown below.

♦ Combination Therapy

Doses may need to be increased or given more frequently when other anticonvulsants (e.g., phenobarbital, phenytoin) are also administered.

♦ Pregnancy

Dose rate requirements may be 100% higher and should be individualized based on plasma concentration measurements.

♦ Children

Dose rate requirements are highest in younger children (0–3 wk) and in children taking other anticonvulsants. A larger proportion of the daily dose may be given at bedtime to avoid breakthrough seizures in the morning.

COMMON TOXICITIES AND ADVERSE REACTIONS

TOXICITY	INCIDENCE	CLINICAL COMMENTS
Dose-Related		
Nystagmus	50%	Overall the incidence of dose-related side effects is 35–50%.
Ataxia	50%	
Diplopia	16%	
Drowsiness	11%	Higher incidence soon after initiation of therapy; higher incidence of neurosensory effects in elderly.
Blurred vision	6%	
Nausea & vomiting	4%	
Paresthesia	3%	
Cardiac conduction disturbances	Rare	Cardiac function should be evaluated in the elderly before carbamazepine is initiated.
Osteomalacia	Uncommon	Symptoms are uncommon; biochemical evidence is common and related to carbamazepine dose and duration; serum calcium and alkaline phosphatase should be periodically measured, especially in patients on longer term, high-dose therapy.
Hypothyroidism	Rare	Although biochemical evidence (lower serum thyroid concentrations) is common, symptoms are rare.
Hypersensitivity		
Skin rashes	2%	Most skin rashes are mildly eczematous and may not require withdrawal of therapy.
Stevens-Johnson syndrome	Rare	
Lupus-like reaction	Rare	

TOXICITY	INCIDENCE	CLINICAL COMMENTS
Idiosyncratic Reactions		
Leukopenia, thrombocytopenia, anemia	2–10%	Leukopenia is transient in 10%, persistent in 2%.
Aplastic anemia	Rare	Blood and platelet counts should be monitored before initiation of therapy and at regular intervals thereafter.
Hepatic Abnormal liver function tests Hepatitis Cholestatic & hepatocellular jaundice	Rare	Liver function tests should be evaluated at baseline and periodic intervals. Liver function test to evaluate for the presence cholestasis, hepatocellular jaundice, and hepatitis.
Nephrotoxicity	Rare	Usually mild and transient.

DRUG INTERACTIONS

DRUG	MECHANISM	CLINICAL COMMENTS
Drugs that Alter Carbamazepine Plasma Concentrations		
Phenytoin Phenobarbital Primidone	Enhanced metabolism by hepatic microsomal enzyme induction	↓ CBZ concentrations, ↑ epoxide concentrations; coadministration with more than one enzyme-inducer ↓ CBZ concentration; ↑ dose rates and ↓ dosing intervals may be required
Propoxyphene Cimetidine Isoniazid Erythromycin Troleandomycin	Inhibition of CBZ metabolism	CBZ dose rates may need to be ↓ if these drugs are given concurrently; plasma concentration monitoring after initiation and discontinuation
Valproic acid	Enzyme inhibition of the epoxide metabolite	Concentrations of CBZ are unchanged and ↑ epoxide concentrations may be evaluated; ↓ in dose rate is probably unnecessary
Effects of Carbamazepine on Other Drugs		
Doxycycline	Induction of hepatic microsomal enzyme activity	↓ half-life; ↑ dose rates may be required for adequate treatment

DRUG	MECHANISM	CLINICAL COMMENTS
Ethosuximide Valproic acid Clonazepam	Enzyme induction	CBZ ↑ dosage requirements of anticonvulsants and more frequent administration may be necessary
Theophylline	Enzyme induction	↓ plasma concentrations and a ↑ theophylline clearance have resulted in loss of asthma control; ↑ theophylline dosage
Warfarin	Induction of hepatic microsomal enzyme activity	Diminished effect of warfarin (shorter prothrombin times)

CLINICAL INTERPRETATION

Carbamazepine SDC data must be interpreted together with the patient's current clinical status, response, and pharmacokinetic considerations. Important factors to consider are:

- Patients receiving carbamazepine together with other antiepileptic drugs may exhibit a therapeutic response between 4 and 8 μg/mL and toxicity between 9 and 12 μg/mL. Patients receiving CBZ alone may respond best to SDC between 8 and 12 μg/mL.

- There are few data available on the effects of various disease states on CBZ disposition. However, because the drug is almost completely metabolized by the liver, its clearance may be decreased by disease of the liver.

- Other concomitant drug therapy

- Age (children have higher reported plasma clearances than adults)

- Pregnancy increases CBZ total body clearance

DIGOXIN

CLINICAL PHARMACOKINETICS
SUMMARY TABLE

SERUM CONCENTRATIONS		
Minimum effective concentration	0.8 ng/mL	
Potentially toxic concentration	> 2.0 ng/mL	
% BIOAVAILABILITY	Tablet	~68%
	Elixir	~77%
	Capsule	~97%
	Intramuscular	~80% (not recommended)
TIME TO PEAK CONCENTRATION	~1 h (tablet)	
TIME TO STEADY-STATE	5–8.0 d (normal)	
	22.0 d (anuric)	
HALF-LIFE (T½)		
Adults	40 h (normal)	
	120 h (anuric)	
Premature infants	60 h	
Neonates	35–45 h	
Infants	18–33 h	
Children	12–24 h	
VOLUME OF DISTRIBUTION		
Adults	~500–600 L	7.4 L/kg nl renal function
Children	Variable (greater than adults on a L/kg basis)	
CLEARANCE		
Total body clearance		
Adults	188 mL/min/1.73m^2 (nl), 45 mL/min/1.73m^2 (severe renal impairment)	
Children		
Neonates	30–40 mL/min/1.73m^2	
Infants, children	130–190 mL/min/1.73m^2	
Dialysis clearance	Insignificant	Plasma is almost completely cleared of digoxin during dialysis, however, most of the drug is in the peripheral tissues and therefore the total body stores are insignificantly affected.
% PROTEIN-BOUND	25%	
% EXCRETED RENALLY UNCHANGED	75% (normal renal function)	
ELIMINATION RATE CONSTANT		
Adults	0.018 h^{-1} (normal)	
	0.007 h^{-1} (anuric)	
Children	Age-dependent	
MAJOR ROUTE OF ELIMINATION	Renal excretion	
ACTIVE METABOLITES	Digoxigenin digitoxose	
	Digoxigenin mono-digitoxose	

THERAPEUTIC DRUG MONITORING

GENERAL GUIDELINES

Samples for routine analysis are obtained in standard vacutainer tubes (red top, no anticoagulant) with care taken to avoid hemolysis. The timing of the sample is particularly important. Following oral or parenteral administration, digoxin SDC decay curves demonstrate a multiphasic distribution that includes an initial rapid disposition phase extending up to 8h after drug administration by either route. This phase, which is frequently referred to as the distribution phase, is most notable with the IV dosage form. Therefore, the patient's SDC must be determined beyond digoxin's distribution phase for reliable interpretation. To evaluate maintenance doses, the patient should be at steady-state (3 to 5 elimination half-lives) when sample is collected. Serum samples should not be drawn for at least 8h, and preferably not for 12h, after oral or IV dose administration if the misleading influences of this slow disposition phase are to be avoided.

SAMPLE COLLECTION

- 8–24 h after administration dose

CLINICAL MONITORING PARAMETERS

- Electrolytes
- Renal Function
- Hepatic Function
- Heart Rate

THERAPEUTICS

USUAL DOSING PARAMETERS

PATIENT GROUP	INITIAL DOSE µg/kg	DAILY MAINTENANCE µg/kg/d	APPROXIMATE T½ NORMAL RENAL FUNCTION
Pediatric			
Neonates	15–18 (IV)	10 (PO)	~35-45 h
Infants	20–25 (IV)	15 (PO)	~8-25 h
Children	20–40 (IV)	8–10 (PO)	~35h
Adults			
Normal renal function	15 (IV) for arrhythmia (AF) 10 for CHF	3.5–5.0 (PO)	1.6 d
Severe renal failure	5–8 (IV)	Varies with renal function	

CLINICAL COMMENTS

♦ Initial and maintenance dosage recommendations in pediatric patients vary widely. Previous literature reports suggest that dosages substantially higher than those used in adults (µg/kg) were necessary. More recent data indicate that lower dosages are adequate to achieve desired therapeutic effects.

♦ Digoxin dosages in adults should be based on both lean body weight and renal function. In older adults, lean body weight as well as renal function are decreased. In pregnant patients both parameters are usually increased.

♦ The doses listed are to be taken only as approximate starting doses. **Oral digoxin loading doses will normally be 20% higher than IV doses.** Further doses (remainder of loading dose or maintenance dose) should be carefully titrated to patient response and SDC.

- Careful attention must be paid to each patient's renal function when determining dosage.

- In adults with renal failure, maintenance dose regimen should be adjusted to individual patient requirements. The dosing interval for each patient should be selected individually based on age, clinical response, and renal function.

- Bioavailability of digoxin products is highly variable. For example, bioavailability of the Lanoxin tablet is approximately 68%, Lanoxin elixir is approximately 77%, and Lanoxicap is 95–100%.

- Generic products should be avoided.

- The initiation of quinidine therapy in a patient receiving digoxin who is at steady-state may result in an increase in serum digoxin concentration. Careful monitoring of serum digoxin concentrations is recommended in such a situation.

COMMON TOXICITIES AND ADVERSE REACTIONS

TOXICITY	INCIDENCE	CLINICAL COMMENTS
Cardiac Effects		Cardiac effects may be cited as the most frequent initial manifestation of digitalis toxicity. However, these data usually accumulated from retrospective studies, may reflect the fact that cardiotoxicity is more likely to cause patients to seek medical attention or is more likely to be directly attributed to digitalis therapy than CNS or GI effects.
Premature ventricular contractions	41–50%	
Atrioventricular (AV) junctional rhythms	17%	
AV block (1^0)*	8–15%	
AV block (2^0 or 3^0)*	8–15%	
Supraventricular tachycardia	8–14%	
Ventricular tachycardia	11%	
Atrial fibrillation	10–14%	
* Incidence in "toxic" pts.		
Central Nervous System Effects		CNS effects are among the most common toxicities identified and, along with GI signs/symptoms, the earliest indication of digitalis toxicity. The relative incidence may depend upon whether the onset of toxicity is abrupt or gradual as well as whether the symptoms/signs are documented by unsolicited patient report or specific.
Fatigue	10–95%	
Weakness	6–82%	
Visual symptoms	11–95%	
Dizziness	10–59%	
Headache	7–45%	
Insomnia/sleep disturbance	10–54%	
Gastrointestinal Effects		GI symptoms/signs are probably the result of a CNS action of digitalis. They are among the most commonly recognized/identified side effects of digitalis.
Anorexia	~70%	
Nausea	~70%	
Diarrhea	6–41%	
Abdominal pain/cramps	1–65%	
Psychic Disorders	1–65%	

DRUG INTERACTIONS

DRUG	MECHANISM	CLINICAL COMMENTS
Aluminum-containing antacids Charcoal Dietary fiber Kaolin-pectin	Intraluminal intestinal binding of digoxin and ↓ absorption	Nonabsorbable drugs or dietary constituents may bind digoxin in the GI tract, preventing absorption and ↓ SDC. **Note:** Kaopectate is most significant; correct by spacing doses at least 2–4 h apart
Tetracycline, broad-spectrum antibiotics	Alteration of intestinal bacterial flora; ↓ intraluminal metabolism of digoxin to reduced dihydrodigoxin	Clinical significance is difficult to predict; only occurs in 10% of patients. This results in an ↑ in SDC of digoxin
Propantheline bromide, diphenoxylate/atropine	↑ absorption	Monitor for ↑ digoxin effect
Metoclopramide	↓ absorption	Monitor for ↓ digoxin effect
Phenobarbital, phenylbutazone, rifampin	↑ hepatic microsomal metabolism of digoxin; ↓ t½	Digoxin dose may need to be ↑ to account for ↑ elimination
Calcium preparations	Possibly ↑ inotropic effect	Avoid concomitant use
Cholestyramine	Intraluminal binding; ↓ absorption, enterohepatic recycling	Administration of digoxin and cholestyramine should be separated by at least 2 h
Diuretics (non-potassium-sparing)	Diuretic-induced hypokalemia	An ↑ incidence of digitalis toxicity (specifically cardiac adverse effects) in patients concurrently receiving potassium-depleting diuretics; potassium replacement is usually required
Calcium channel-blocking agents (diltiazem, nifedipine, verapamil)	↓ renal and/or extrarenal clearance	Concomitant use of each of the 3 available calcium channel-blocking agents has been associated with ↑ in the serum digoxin concentrations similar to that observed with quinidine
Quinidine	↓ tissue binding; ↓ total body clearance	Concomitant use of quinidine may result in a 50–100% ↑ in the steady-state serum digoxin concentration

CLINICAL INTERPRETATION

- SDC data must be interpreted together with the patient's current clinical status, response, and pharmacokinetic considerations.

- SDC should be drawn 8–24 h after drug administration or immediately before administration of next oral dose for proper interpretation.

Factors Affecting Myocardial Sensitivity	Digoxin Effect
♦ Severe congestive heart failure	Increased
♦ Hypothyroidism	Increased
♦ Hypomagnesemia	Increased
♦ Hypercalcemia	Increased
♦ Pulmonary heart disease (e.g., cor pulmonale)	Increased
♦ Acute myocardial ischemia	Increased
♦ Acute myocardial infarction	Increased
♦ Acute myocarditis	Increased
♦ Cardiomyopathies	Increased
♦ Valvular lesions	Increased
♦ Hyperthyroidism	Decreased

Factors Affecting Serum Concentrations	Digoxin SDC
♦ Renal disease	Increased
♦ Hepatic disease	Increased
♦ Severe congestive heart failure	Increased
♦ Concomitant drug therapy: quinidine	Increased
♦ Spironolactone	Increased
♦ Liquid antacids	Decreased
♦ Kaolin-pectin preparations	Decreased
♦ Malabsorption	Decreased
♦ Reduced GI motility	Increased
♦ Fast dissolution rate	Increased
♦ Increased GI motility	Decreased
♦ Sprue	Decreased
♦ Small intestine resection (excluding jejunoileal bypass)	Decreased
♦ Radiation to abdomen	Decreased
♦ Hyperthyroidism (↑ Vd)	Decreased
♦ Hypothyroidism (↓ Vd)	Increased
♦ Slow dissolution rate	Decreased
♦ Poor bioavailability	Decreased

DIGITOXIN

CLINICAL PHARMACOKINETICS

SUMMARY TABLE

SERUM CONCENTRATIONS		
Minimum effective concentration	15 ng/mL	
Potentially toxic concentration	> 40 ng/mL	
% BIOAVAILABILITY	Tablet	90-100%
	Intravenous	(?)
TIME TO PEAK CONCENTRATION	~1 h (tablet)	
TIME TO STEADY-STATE	~34 d (normal) ~40 d (anuric)	
HALF-LIFE (T½)		
Adults	~163 h (normal) ~192 h (anuric)	
Children	~154 h	
VOLUME OF DISTRIBUTION		
Adults	0.6 L/kg	
Children	Variable (greater than adults on a L/kg basis)	
CLEARANCE		
Total body clearance		
Adults	0.02-0.04 mL/min/kg	
Children	0.09 mL/min/kg	
Dialysis clearance	Insignificant	
% PROTEIN-BOUND	90-95%	
% EXCRETED RENALLY UNCHANGED	15%	
ELIMINATION RATE CONSTANT		
Adults	0.004 h^{-1} (normal) 0.004 h^{-1} (anuric)	
Children	0.005 h^{-1}	
MAJOR ROUTE OF ELIMINATION	hepatic 50-70% renal for metabolites	
ACTIVE METABOLITES	Digoxin Digoxin metabolites	

THERAPEUTIC DRUG MONITORING

GENERAL GUIDELINES

Samples for routine analysis are obtained in standard vacutainer tubes (red top, no anticoagulant) with care taken to avoid hemolysis. The timing of the sample is particularly important. To evaluate maintenance doses, the patient should be at steady-state (3 to 5 elimination half-lives) when sample is collected. Serum samples should not be drawn for at least 4 hours after IV or 6 hours after an oral dose.

SAMPLE COLLECTION

- 4–24 h after administration dose (see above), trough samples preferred

CLINICAL MONITORING PARAMETERS

- Electrolytes
- Renal Function
- Hepatic Function
- Heart Rate

THERAPEUTICS

USUAL DOSING PARAMETERS

PATIENT GROUP	INITIAL DOSE µg/kg	DAILY MAINTE-NANCE µg/kg/d	APPROXIMATE T½ NORMAL HEPATIC/ RENAL FUNCTION
Pediatric			
Premature			*
Neonates	20-30 (PO/IV)	2-4 (PO/IV)	*
Infants	20–40 (PO/IV)	2-4 (PO/IV)	*
Children	20–40 (PO/IV)	3 (PO/IV)	6.4 d
Adults			
Adults	15-25 (PO/IV)	1-2.5 (PO/IV)	7.0 d

* Data not available

CLINICAL COMMENTS

- Initial and maintenance dosage recommendations in pediatric patients vary widely. Previous literature reports suggest that dosages substantially higher than those used in adults (µg/kg) were necessary. More recent data indicate that lower dosages are adequate to achieve desired therapeutic effects.

- Digitoxin dosages in adults should be based on ideal body weight.

- The doses listed are to be taken only as approximate starting doses. Further doses (remainder of loading dose or maintenance dose) should be carefully titrated to patient response and SDC.

- The initiation of quinidine therapy in a patient receiving digitoxin who is at steady-state may result in an increase in serum digitoxin concentration. Careful monitoring of serum digitoxin concentrations is recommended in such a situation.

COMMON TOXICITIES AND ADVERSE REACTIONS

TOXICITY	INCIDENCE	CLINICAL COMMENTS
Cardiac Effects		Cardiac effects are often cited as the most frequent initial manifestation of digitalis toxicity. However, most of this data accumulated from retrospective studies and may reflect the fact that cardiotoxicity is more likely to cause patients to seek medical attention or is more likely to be directly attributed to digitalis therapy than CNS or GI effects.
Premature ventricular contractions	41–50%	
Atrioventricular (AV) junctional rhythms	17%	
AV block (1^0)	8–15%*	
AV block (2^0 or 3^0)	8–15%*	
Supraventricular tachycardia	8–14%	
Ventricular tachycardia	11%	
Atrial fibrillation	10–14%	
* Incidence in "toxic" pts.		
Central Nervous System Effects		CNS effects are among the most common toxicities identified and, along with GI signs/symptoms, the earliest indication of digitalis toxicity. The wide variance in reported incidence may depend upon whether the onset of toxicity is abrupt or gradual as well as whether the symptoms/ signs are documented by unsolicited patient report or by specific questioning.
Fatigue	10–95%	
Weakness	6–82%	
Visual symptoms	11–95%	
Dizziness	10–59%	
Headache	7–45%	
Insomnia/sleep disturbance	10–54%	
Gastrointestinal Effects		GI symptoms/signs are probably the result of a CNS action of digitalis. They are among the most commonly recognized side effects of digitalis.
Anorexia	~70%	
Nausea	~70%	
Diarrhea	6–41%	
Abdominal pain/cramps	1–65%	
Psychic Disorders	1–65%	

DRUG INTERACTIONS

DRUG	MECHANISM	CLINICAL COMMENTS
Aluminum-containing antacids Charcoal Dietary fiber Kaolin-pectin	Intraluminal intestinal binding of digitoxin and ↓ absorption	Nonabsorbable drugs or dietary constituents may bind digitoxin in the GI tract, preventing absorption and ↓ SDC. **Note:** Kaopectate is most significant; correct by spacing doses at least 2–4 h apart.
Propantheline bromide, diphenoxylate/atropine	↑ absorption	Monitor for ↑ digitoxin effect.
Phenobarbital, phenylbutazone, rifampin	↑ hepatic microsomal metabolism of digitoxin; ↓ t½	Digitoxin dose may need to be ↑ to account for ↑ elimination. Watch for toxicity if patient is noncompliant or the interacting drug is discontinued without a decrease in digitoxin dose.
Calcium preparations	Possibly ↑ inotropic effect	Avoid concomitant use.
Colestipol, Cholestyramine	Intraluminal binding; ↓ absorption, enterohepatic recycling	Administration of digitoxin and cholestyramine should be separated by at least 2 h
Calcium channel-blocking agents (diltiazem, nifedipine, verapamil)	Reduces total body Cl and extrarenal Cl of digitoxin	Concomitant use of each of the 3 available calcium channel-blocking agents has been associated with ↑ in the serum digitoxin concentrations similar to that observed with quinidine
Amiodarone, Quinidine	↓ renal & nonrenal Cl concomitant use of quinidine and digitoxin. May result in ↑ plasma digitoxin concentration. Digitoxin dosage should be ↓ as necessary.	Concomitant use of quinidine may result in a 50–100% ↑ in the steady-state serum digitoxin concentration
Aminogutethimide	↑ metabolism of digitoxin	Monitor for ↓ digitoxin effect

CLINICAL INTERPRETATION

- SDC data must be interpreted together with the patient's current clinical status, response, and pharmacokinetic considerations.

- SDC should be drawn 10–24 h after drug administration or immediately before administration of next oral dose for proper interpretation.

Factors Affecting Myocardial Sensitivity	Digitoxin Effect
♦ Severe pulmonary disease	↑
♦ Hypothyroidism	↑
♦ Hyperthyroidism	↓
♦ Acute myocardial infarction	↑
♦ Severe congestive heart failure	↑
♦ Acute myocarditis	↑
♦ Hypomagnesemia	↑
♦ Hypercalcemia	↑
♦ Hypokalemia	↑
♦ Cardiomyopathies	↑
♦ Valvular lesions	↑

Factors Affecting Serum Concentrations	Digitoxin SDC
♦ Severe congestive heart failure	↑
♦ Quinidine	↑
♦ Amiodarone	↑
♦ Spironolactone	↑
♦ Calcium-channel blockers	↑
♦ Propantheline	↑
♦ Biliary fistulas	↓
♦ Charcoal	↓
♦ Dietary fibers	↓
♦ Liquid antacids	↓
♦ Kaolin-pectin preparations	↓
♦ Phenobarbital	↓
♦ Phenylbutazone	↓
♦ Rifampin	↓
♦ Aminoglutethimide	↓

GENTAMICIN/
TOBRAMYCIN

CLINICAL PHARMACOKINETICS

SUMMARY TABLE

SERUM CONCENTRATIONS		
Severe systemic infections (Minimum effective concentrations)	Peak concentration Trough concentration	6–10 μg/mL 0.5–<2 μg/mL
Potentially toxic concentrations	Peak concentration Trough concentration	>12–15 μg/mL >2 μg/mL
TIME TO PEAK CONCENTRATION	IM administration IV administration	0.5–1 h Immediately post-infusion
TIME TO STEADY-STATE	Variable, 10–15 h in normal renal function	Steady-state is generally achieved in 4–5 half-lives
HALF-LIFE (T½)		
Normal renal function	Average $S_{cr} \leq 1.5$ mg/dL $CL_{cr} \geq 100$ mL/min/1.73m^2	2 h 0.5–15 h 0.5–8 h
Age	Neonates Children Adults ≤ 30 yr old Adults > 30 yr old	2–9 h 0.5–3 h 0.5–3 h 1.5–15 h
Entire range of renal function		0.7–70 h
VOLUME OF DISTRIBUTION		
Adults	Dehydration Normal fluid status Increased extracellular fluid	0.05–0.15 L/kg 0.15–0.25 L/kg 0.25–0.70 L/kg
Children Neonates		0.07–0.70 L/kg 0.20–0.70 L/kg
CLEARANCE		
Total body clearance	Normal S_{cr} (≤1.5 mg/dL) Abnormal S_{cr} (≥1.5 mg/dL) $CL_{cr} \geq 100$ mL/min	1.33 ± 0.61 mL/min/kg 0.53 ± 0.35 mL/min/kg 1.51 ± 0.60 mL/min/kg
Dialysis clearance	Hemodialysis 6–hr hemodialysis Peritoneal dialysis	30–60 mL/min 40–60% Less effective in removing amino-glycosides
% PROTEIN-BOUND		0–30%
% EXCRETED RENALLY UNCHANGED	Unchanged	85–95%
MAJOR ROUTE OF ELIMINATION		Glomerular filtration; ~99% of dose renally excreted unchanged
ACTIVE METABOLITES		None known

THERAPEUTIC DRUG MONITORING

GENERAL GUIDELINES

- The interpatient variability of gentamicin/tobramycin pharmacokinetics, the seriousness of gram-negative infections, and the risk of toxicity require that patients receiving these aminoglycosides be monitored closely. Both peak and trough concentrations should be monitored closely and dosages adjusted to attain desired SDC.

- Methods, e.g. those described by Zaske, allow the clinician to calculate the dose and dosing interval from the SDC-time data, although the frequency of monitoring should be determined for each patient. Monitoring is indicated.

- Assess the adequacy of therapy based on therapeutic guidelines for a specific pathogen, site of infection, and clinical condition of the patient.

- To prevent excessively high SDC and reduce the risk of toxicity

- Renal function changes

- Changes in volume

- Dosage and/or dosing interval changes

SAMPLE COLLECTION

Peak	IM	60 min after injection
	IV	30 min after a 30–min infusion or immediately after a 60–min infusion
Trough	IV	Immediately before administration of subsequent dose (under steady-state condition)
		These values influenced by the patient's hydration status, may indicate changing renal function; resolution or worsening of the infection; there is an additive risk for toxicity

CLINICAL COMMENTS

- Both peak and trough concentrations should be measured over the same dosing interval.

- Sampling is often done prior to attainment of steady-state to help prevent toxicity and to ensure therapeutic efficacy.

- The use of heparinized tubes to collect specimens for aminoglycosides analysis is controversial. Until the controversy is resolved, heparinized tubes should not be used to collect specimens.

- High concentrations of beta-lactam antibiotics (penicillins) inactivate aminoglycosides in vivo and in vitro. Specimens containing a beta-lactam antibiotic in addition to an aminoglycoside should be either assayed immediately using a rapid method or stored frozen.

CLINICAL MONITORING PARAMETERS

- Blood urea nitrogen (BUN)
- Concomitant antibiotics and other potentially ototoxic or nephrotoxic drugs
- Cultures and sensitivities
- Fluid intake and output (I/O)
- Hemoglobin/hematocrit
- Maximum body temperature per 24–hr period
- Patient weight
- Serum creatinine (S_{cr})
- White blood cell count (WBC) with differential
- X-rays

THERAPEUTICS

USUAL DOSING PARAMETERS

PATIENT GROUP	INITIAL DOSE	DAILY MAINTENANCE	APPROXIMATE T½ NORMAL RENAL FUNCTION
Pediatric		1–2 mg/kg q 4–8 h	0.5–3 h
Dehydrated	0.75–1.5 mg/kg		
Normal hydration	1–2 mg/kg		
Increased extracellular fluid	1.5–2.5 mg/kg		
Normal renal function		1–2 mg/kg q 4–8 h	0.5–3 h
Abnormal renal function		variable	variable
Neonates	2–2.5 mg/kg	2–2.5 mg/kg q 8–24 h	2–9 h
Adult		1–2 mg/kg q 6–12 h	
Dehydrated	0.75–1.5 mg/kg		
Normal hydration	1–2 mg/kg		
Increased extracellular fluid	1.5–2.5 mg/kg		
Normal renal function		1–2 mg/kg q 6–12 h	0.5–3 h (<30 yr old) 1.5–15 h (>30 yr old)
Abnormal renal function		Adjust according to renal function	0.7–43 h

CLINICAL COMMENTS

- These are suggested starting dosages. They may exceed manufacturer's recommendations and reflect opinions of usual dosages required to achieve therapeutic SDC in patients with serious infections and normal renal function. The monitoring of SDC is required. In neonates the dosage is based on gestational age and body weight.

- Dosing intervals should be adjusted based on patient response, SDC, and renal function.

- Administer in 2 or 3 divided doses. In patients with abnormal renal function, adjust dosage according to renal status and SDC.

- If administered intravenously, infuse over 30–60 min.

- Usual therapeutic range will be dependent on infecting organism, site of infection, immunological status of the patient, and severity of infection.

- Dosage requirements will vary depending on birth-weight and maturity; SDC should be monitored.

- With abnormal renal function, half-life is quite variable.

COMMON TOXICITIES AND ADVERSE REACTIONS

TOXICITY	RISK FACTORS	CLINICAL COMMENTS
Ototoxicity (Incidence: 1–2%)	Concomitant ototoxic drugs Prior exposure to aminoglycosides Duration of treatment > 10–15 days Cumulative dose Total daily dose Sustained peak concentrations > 12–15 μg/mL Sustained trough concentrations > 2 μg/mL Age > 60 years Renal insufficiency Dialysis	Ototoxicity is primarily cochlear but vestibular dysfunction also occurs. Most studies demonstrated the incidence of decreased hearing to be 2–10% by audiometry. Overt clinical toxicity is only about 1–2%. Auditory dysfunction is usually in the higher frequencies, but conversational hearing loss can occur. It is usually bilateral and permanent. Vestibular dysfunction usually manifests as slight vertigo or tinnitus, although acute Meniere's syndrome can occur. It is usually permanent. However, patients can overcome the dysfunction by compensatory mechanisms. They have greater difficulty ambulating in the dark.
Nephrotoxicity (Incidence: 2–10%)	Concomitant nephrotoxic drugs Prior exposure to aminoglycosides Total dose received Mean peak plasma concentrations > 12–15 μg/mL Elevated peak plasma concentrations (>15 μg/mL) Sustained trough concentration > 2 μg/mL Volume depletion Age > 60 years Renal insufficiency	Most studies demonstrated toxicity by an increase in serum creatinine and BUN. Overt nonoliguric renal failure occurs uncommonly, provided drug accumulation does not occur. Typical findings include a decreased glomerular filtration rate and impaired urinary concentrating ability. This usually occurs at least five days after initiating therapy. A Fanconi-like syndrome may occur.

TOXICITY	RISK FACTORS	CLINICAL COMMENTS
Neuro-muscular blockade (Incidence: Infrequent)	Concomitant administration of neuromuscular blocking agents and anesthetics Inpatients with hypocalcemia Myasthenia gravis High SDC in newborns When administered intraperitoneally or rapid IV injection	Blockade is usually competitive, although a noncompetitive block may occur. Respiratory depression and apnea may be quickly reversed by administering calcium or anticholinesterase.
Other Adverse Effects		
Headache and Nausea (Incidence: < 1%)	Unknown	Reported reaction but of questionable association.
Abnormal liver function tests (Incidence: Rare)	Unknown	This reaction has been reported but is not definitely associated with therapy.
Teratogenicity (Incidence: Infrequent)	Unknown	Not systematically studied... potential for ototoxicity and nephrotoxicity.
Tachycardia (Incidence: Infrequent)	Unknown	Questionable.
Allergic or Hypersensitivity Reactions (Incidence: 1–3%)	Possibly the length of the therapy	Rash, eosinophilia, and drug fever have been reported with incidence varying from 0.1% to 11%. However, the overall incidence may vary with the type of observation.

DRUG INTERACTIONS

DRUG	MECHANISM	CLINICAL COMMENTS
Amphotericin B	Synergistic nephrotoxicity may be exhibited	Patients receiving both agents concurrently should be closely monitored for renal function deterioration
Cephalosporins	Synergistic nephrotoxicity may be exhibited	May occur primarily with cephaloridine and cephalothin; closely monitor patient's renal function
Clindamycin	Likelihood of aminoglycoside nephrotoxicity which may be enhanced	Monitor patient's renal function carefully
Dimenhydrinate	Aminoglycoside ototoxicity may be masked	Monitor patient's cochlear and vestibular function carefully
Ethacrynic acid/furosemide	Aminoglycoside ototoxicity and nephrotoxicity may be potentiated	Monitor patient for ototoxicity and nephrotoxicity carefully
Heparin (>5–10 units/mL)	Possible chemical complex formation, usually reversible	Aminoglycoside concentration determinations may be erroneously low
Methoxyflurane	May include additive or synergistic nephrotoxicity	Monitor patient's renal function closely
Semisynthetic penicillins (carbenicillin, ticarcillin, piperacillin) and other beta-lactam antibiotics	Chemical complex formation, reversible	Aminoglycoside concentration determinations may be falsely low; may result in microbiologically inactive compounds; greatest effect may be seen with gentamicin and carbenicillin
Neuromuscular blocking agents and skeletal muscle relaxants	Aminoglycoside-induced neuromuscular blockade may be synergistic	Concurrent administration should be avoided since neuromuscular blockade may be enhanced; anticholinesterase agents may reverse the blockade

OTHER

A number of other agents may interact with gentamicin/tobramycin, including vancomycin, polymyxins, furosemide, cisplatin, and general anesthesia

CLINICAL INTERPRETATION

Gentamicin/tobramycin SDC data should be interpreted in the context of the patient's current clinical status, response, and other pharmacotherapeutic considerations. There are a number of factors that potentially alter the pharmacokinetics, therapeutics, and SDC of gentamicin/tobramycin. These factors must be taken into consideration when determining monitoring frequency and the clinical interpretation of a gentamicin/tobramycin blood level. They include:

MAY REQUIRE AN INCREASE IN DAILY DOSE

- Extremely burned patients
- Markedly obese individuals
- Patients with cystic fibrosis
- Patients with ascites
- Congestive heart failure
- Age (neonates have large apparent volume of distribution)
- Concomitant drug therapy: heparin (in vivo inactivation unlikely); high concentrations of certain penicillins, (e.g., carbenicillin, ticarcillin, and possibly ampicillin)----in vivo inactivation significant only in patients with renal failure

MAY REQUIRE A DECREASE IN DAILY DOSE

- Premature or underweight newborns
- Patients with reduced renal function
- Elderly patients
- Conditions associated with decreased volume of distribution (dehydration, etc.)

OTHER CONSIDERATIONS

- Recent myocardial infarction: initial SDC may be reduced (increased volume of distribution and prolonged elimination half-life)
- Collection tubes (see note in introduction)
- Peritonitis

LIDOCAINE

CLINICAL PHARMACOKINETICS
SUMMARY TABLE

SERUM CONCENTRATIONS	Minimum effective concentration	1.5 µg/mL
	Potentially toxic concentration	>5 µg/mL
% BIOAVAILABILITY	Intramuscular	100%
	Intravenous	100%
	Oral	25–50%
	Rectal	30–100%
TIME TO PEAK CONCENTRATION	After loading dose at the end of the IV infusion	
TIME TO STEADY-STATE	Normal patients (without loading dose)	6–12 h
	Loading dose	0.5–1.5 h
HALF-LIFE (T½)	Cardiac failure	2–6 h
	Cirrhosis	5 h
	Normals	1–2.3 h
	Uremia	1.3 h
VOLUME OF DISTRIBUTION	Cardiac failure	62 L/1.73 m^2
	Cirrhosis	162 L/1.73 m^2
	Normals	130 L/1.73 m^2
	Uremia	84 L/1.73 m^2
CLEARANCE		
Plasma (normal)		0.54–144 L/min
Dialysis		27 mL/min
% PROTEIN-BOUND	Concentration dependent	~70%
	Uremia	80–90%
	Myocardial infarction	60–90%
% EXCRETED RENALLY UNCHANGED	<10% at low urinary pH	
MAJOR ROUTE OF ELIMINATION	Hepatic	
ACTIVE METABOLITES	Monoethylglycinexylidide	Potency similar to lidocaine's
	Glycinexylidide	Potency 25% of lidocaine's

THERAPEUTIC DRUG MONITORING

GENERAL GUIDELINES

- The clinical efficacy of lidocaine can be measured only retrospectively, but monitoring of plasma lidocaine concentrations may be of value in maintaining adequate plasma concentrations while avoiding severe drug toxicity. Generally, the patient should be at steady-state (3–5 elimination half-lives) to ensure reliable interpretation of a SDC result.

INDICATIONS FOR MONITORING

- Anytime lidocaine toxicity is suspected
- Anytime ventricular arrhythmias occur during administration of lidocaine, in order to determine whether ineffectiveness may be due to pharmacokinetic or targeted organ factors
- Twelve hours after the initiation of lidocaine therapy for ventricular arrhythmia prophylaxis following acute myocardial infarction, and every 24h as long as lidocaine is administered
- Every 12h in patients with congestive heart failure or hepatic insufficiency
- If other drugs known to affect lidocaine clearance are administered concomitantly (e.g., propranolol, cimetidine)

CLINICAL MONITORING PARAMETERS

- Blood pressure
- CNS status
- Electrolytes
- IV infusion rate
- I & O
- ECG

THERAPEUTICS

USUAL DOSING PARAMETERS

PATIENT GROUP	INITIAL DOSE	DAILY MAINTENANCE	APPROXIMATE T½ NORMAL RENAL FUNCTION
Pediatric	1-5 mg/kg	20–40 μg/kg/min (total dose of 5 mg/kg)	Insufficient data
Adult			
Normal (adults)	200–300 mg	1.5-3.0 mg/min	~1.5h
Congestive heart failure	110–160 mg	0.9-1.8 mg/min	~2h
Cirrhosis	200–300 mg	0.9-1.8 mg/min	~5h

CLINICAL COMMENTS

- Constant infusion or repeated injections administered at a rate not to exceed 50 mg/min.
- Treatment of breakthrough arrhythmias (adult): administer an additional 50 mg bolus over 2-5 min and increase infusion in increments of 1 mg/min (e.g., 2 mg/min increases to 3 mg/min).
- Administer loading doses either by constant infusion or by repeated slow IV injection.
- Lidocaine dosing in pediatrics has not been adequately evaluated. The above dosing guidelines are based on clinical experience.

COMMON TOXICITIES AND ADVERSE REACTIONS

- Adverse effects tend to occur more commonly in older patients and those with acute myocardial infarction, congestive heart failure, or low body weight.

- Most commonly encountered lidocaine toxicities occur during bolus administration. Administer bolus infusion slowly (over 1–2 min) to allow for adequate distribution.

TOXICITIES	INCIDENCE	CLINICAL COMMENTS
Cardiovascular System Hypotension Arrhythmias Asystole	Rare	Adverse effects tend to occur more commonly in older patients as well as those with acute myocardial infarction, congestive heart failure, or low body weight. Most commonly encountered lidocaine toxicities occur during bolus administration. Administer bolus infusion slowly (over 1–2 min) to allow for adequate distribution.
Central Nervous System Dizziness Drowsiness Euphoria Nausea Paresthesias Tinnitus	Most common	These adverse reactions may not relate to plasma concentrations outside of the therapeutic range after rapid IV bolus. May reduce the incidence of these adverse reactions by administering the loading dose as a slow infusion.
Agitation Coma Confusion Dysarthria Seizures	Rare	Generally related to concentrations > 5 μg/mL. Recommend discontinuation of lidocaine until adverse reaction resolves and plasma concentration returns to the therapeutic range.

TOXICITIES	INCIDENCE	CLINICAL COMMENTS
Neuromuscular System	Relatively common	Muscle twitching
Respiratory System	Rare	Respiratory depression
Others Anaphylactic shock Exfoliative dermatitis	Rare	

DRUG INTERACTIONS

DRUG	MECHANISM	CLINICAL COMMENTS
Antiepileptic drugs (e.g., phenytoin and phenobarbital)	↑ clearance	Probably of limited clinical significance; SDC of antiepileptics may be ↓ by ~10%
Cimetidine	↓ clearance	May ↑ lidocaine toxicity
Glucagon	↑ clearance	Clinical significance unknown
Isoproterenol	↑ clearance	Clinical significance unknown
Metoprolol	↓ clearance	May ↑ lidocaine toxicity
Norepinephrine	↓ clearance	Clinical significance unknown
Phenobarbital	Additive depressant effect on respiratory center	Clinical significance unknown Clinical significance reported in animals only
Phenytoin	Additive cardiac depressant effect	Possible cause of sinoatrial arrest in one patient; clinical significance unknown
Propranolol	↓ clearance	May ↑ lidocaine toxicity

CLINICAL INTERPRETATION

- Total lidocaine SDCs may continue to rise in patients with myocardial infarction, never reaching a steady-state level. However, the rise in free drug concentration is less than the rise in total lidocaine concentration. May be the result of increased lidocaine protein binding. This is probably due to increased alpha$_1$-acid glycoprotein levels in myocardial infarction patients.
- SDC data must be interpreted together with the patient's current clinical status, response, and pharmacokinetic considerations.
- Only limited data are available for children.
- Conditions that influence or change SDC of alpha$_1$-acid glycoprotein will alter unbound concentrations of lidocaine.

Factors Affecting Serum Lidocaine Concentrations

	CLINICAL COMMENTS
Alterations in protein binding	↑ plasma protein binding seen primarily in cancer, cardiac surgery, chronic renal failure, epilepsy (treated), increasing age, myocardial infarction
	↓ plasma protein binding may be clinically significant with acidosis, heparin, hepatic cirrhosis (variable), neonates, nephrotic syndrome (variable), oral contraceptives, quinidine bupivacaine, disopyramide, total lidocaine concentration
Cardiac failure	↓ volume of distribution and clearance can result in ↑ plasma concentrations
Cirrhosis	Marked ↓ in hepatic enzyme activity and liver blood flow can result in ↑ plasma concentration
Drugs (e.g., propranolol, metoprolol, cimetidine)	↑ lidocaine SDC
Vacutainer effect	Can cause spuriously low plasma concentrations by as much as 30% due to binding

LITHIUM

CLINICAL PHARMACOKINETICS
SUMMARY TABLE

SERUM CONCENTRATIONS	
Minimum effective concentrations	
Mania	1.0–1.5 mEq/L
Prophylaxis against mania	0.6–1.2 mEq/L
Potentially toxic concentration	>1.5 mEq/L
% BIOAVAILABILITY	
Regular preparations and liquid	>95%
Slow release	>85%
TIME TO PEAK CONCENTRATION	1–2h (4–5 for slow release)
TIME TO STEADY-STATE	5 (3–10) d (i.e., 4–5 times the half-life)
HALF-LIFE (T½)	
Adults	24 (18–36) h
Children	<adults
VOLUME OF DISTRIBUTION	
Adults	
Total body weight	0.8 (0.5–0.9) L/kg
Central	(0.20–0.25) L/kg
Geriatrics	
Total body weight	~0.7(0.5–1.0) L/kg
Central	(0.20–0.25) L/kg
CLEARANCE	
Total body clearance	
Normal renal function	15–30 mL/min
Compromised renal function	~20% of creatinine clearance
Dialysis clearance	
Hemodialysis	50 mL/min
Peritoneal dialysis	13–15 mL/min
% PROTEIN-BOUND	None
% EXCRETED RENALLY UNCHANGED	95%
ELIMINATION RATE CONSTANT	
Adults	0.029 (0.019–0.039) L/h
Children	> adults
MAJOR ROUTE OF ELIMINATION	Renal excretion
ACTIVE METABOLITES	None

THERAPEUTIC DRUG MONITORING

GENERAL GUIDELINES

- ♦ Generally, the patient should be at steady-state (3–5 elimination half-lives) when sample is collected to ensure reliable interpretation of a SDC result.
- ♦ If only one measurement is going to be made, then a trough concentration provides the best guide for dosage adjustment.

PRE-LITHIUM SCREENING	ASSESSMENT
History and Physical Examination	
Age	Dosing parameter
Height	Dosing parameter
Weight	Dosing parameter
ECG (Over 40 yr of age)	Cardiac function
Laboratory	
Serum creatinine	Renal function
BUN	Fluid status & renal function
Serum electrolytes	Fluid & electrolyte status
Sodium	
Potassium	
Calcium	
Phosphate	
Lithium level	Assure starting lithium concentration
Thyroid function	Baseline
T3	
T4 Index	
TSH	
Complete Blood Count	
WBC	Baseline
Urinalysis	
Specific gravity	Renal, fluid, & electrolyte status
Osmolality	

SAMPLE COLLECTION

INDICATION	WHEN TO SAMPLE
Initial Monitoring	
12-hr post LithoBid loading dose (Pepin[1] method)	12h after LithoBid loading dose
24-hr post test dose (Cooper[2] method)	24h after 600-mg test dose
Series of samples for T½ (Perry[3] method)	12, 18, 24, 36, & 48 h after test dose
Resampling	
Assess side effects	Any time >8h after last dose
Dosing stabilization and adjustment	12h after last dose at steady-state
After a dose change	Wait about 5 half-lives, then resample 12h after last dose
Altered clinical state (renal, fluid & electrolytes, drug interactions)	12h after last dose
Pregnancy	12h level after last dose at weekly intervals
Psychiatric relapse	12h level after last dose; also obtain serum creatinine level

1. Pepin SM, Baker DE, Nance KS et al. Lithium dosage calculation from age, sex, height, weight, and serum creatinine. Presented at the 15th annual ASHP Midyear Clinical Meeting, San Francisco, CA: 1980 Dec. 9.

2. Cooper TB, Bergner P-EE, Simpson GM. The 24-hour serum lithium level as a prognosticator of dosage requirements. Am J Psychiatry. 1973;130:601–603.

3. Perry PJ, Prince RA, Alexander B et al. Prediction of lithium maintenance doses using a single point prediction protocol. J Clin Psychopharmacol. 1983;3:13–17.

Collection Procedure for 12h Standard Lithium Level

Laboratory usually requires 5 mL blood, drawn into a standard red-top serum tube or a heparinized tube, to allow for duplicate determination

- Check to see that patient has not received morning dose lithium
- Draw level at specified time and record to the minute when sample was obtained
- Inform nurse when phlebotomy is completed
- Centrifuge at 2500 RPM for 10 min
- Avoid hemolysis
- Refrigerate until analysis (stable 1 wk at room temperature once removed from the clot)
- Series of urine collection for lithium (Norman method)

CLINICAL COMMENTS

- Even though lithium has not been approved by the FDA for use in children under the age of 12, experience in juvenile manic-depressive illness has demonstrated response and side-effect patterns similar to those seen in adults.

- When other treatments have failed, lithium may be justified for treatment in children. Because of its potential for adverse developmental effects in bone, lithium should be held in reserve. Larger volumes of distribution by percentage of body weight, shorter half-lives, and faster clearances are anticipated in the child.

- The renal function and aging of the patient affects the clearance of lithium. As GFR decreases, clearance of lithium is proportionally reduced.

- Gender appears to have little if any effect on the excretion of lithium. Pregnancy, however, may increase lithium clearance significantly (by 50–100%) because of the greater GFR. Lithium clearance returns to pre-pregnancy values immediately upon delivery.

- Even though marijuana may decrease lithium clearance, cigarette smoking has not been shown to affect lithium pharmacokinetics.

- Burn patients eliminate lithium at an increased rate. Loss from eschar and increases in renal elimination should be anticipated. Fluid and electrolyte fluctuations may preclude the use of lithium in burn patients, however.

- Hemodialysis increases lithium clearance about 50 mL/min. In chronic lithium intoxication there may be a rebound in SDC immediately after hemodialysis due to the movement of lithium from intracellular water to serum.

- Peritoneal dialysis was used for 70h in a chronically intoxicated patient (beginning lithium level = 4.6 mEq/L, ending lithium level = 0.5 mEq/L). This method added 13–15 mL/min to the patient's renal lithium clearance. Rebound was not observed due to the slower rate of lithium extraction.

- Genetics may play a role in transporting lithium. Monozygotic twins had similar ratios of serum-to-RBC lithium levels; dizygotic twins did not.

- Retention of lithium in low-sodium diets can drastically affect lithium clearance. However, this does not preclude the use of lithium in sodium-restricted patients if careful monitoring practices are followed.

CLINICAL MONITORING PARAMETERS

- Renal function
- Thyroid function
- CBC with differential

THERAPEUTICS

USUAL DOSING PARAMETERS

PATIENT GROUP	INITIAL DOSE	DAILY MAINTENANCE	APPROXIMATE T½ NORMAL RENAL FUNCTION
Adult	Only with slow-release formulations 30 mg/kg daily in divided dose	900 mg/d ↑ gradually until patient is in the therapeutic range Usual daily dose requirements are 900–1500 mg/d	24 h

CLINICAL COMMENTS

- Regardless of the way in which the initial daily dosage of lithium is determined, follow-up monitoring and dosage adjustments will be necessary. A steady-state 12h post-dose standard lithium level can be used to calculate an apparent lithium clearance. Based upon this value, a proportional increase or decrease in the daily lithium dosage can be made to maintain the patient's lithium concentration within the desired range.

Product Formulation

Lithium carbonate	8.12 mEq	Per 300 mg
Lithium citrate liquid	8.12 mEq	Per 5 mL
Slow release lithium carbonate	8.12 mEq	Per 300 mg
LithoBid	12.18 mEq	Per 450 mg

Management of Lithium Intoxication	Tests
Gastric lavage (for acute ingestion)	Serum lithium concentration
Supportive treatment	Chest X-ray film
Fluid and electrolyte correction	Serum creatinine level
Maintain kidney function	Serum electrolyte levels
± infection prophylaxis (avoid aspiration)	Blood pressure
Support blood pressure and respiration	Respiration rate
Increase elimination	
Wait for patient's kidneys to eliminate the drug if clinically possible; or consider enhancing elimination	

Methods of Enhancing Lithium Elimination	Expected Increase in Lithium Clearance
Hemodialysis (+50 mL/min)	+500%
Peritoneal dialysis (+15 mL/min)	+100%
Theophylline or aminophylline	+ 50%
Osmotic diuretics	+ 25%
Recline patient	+ 30%

COMMON TOXICITIES AND ADVERSE REACTIONS

TOXICITY	INCIDENCE	CLINICAL COMMENTS
Cardiac		Cardiac assessment. Caution in patients with pre-existing cardiopathy. Periodic ECG monitoring suggested for serious arrhythmias. Reduce dosage or discontinue lithium.
ECG changes	20–30% benign	
T-wave reduced		
Arrhythmias	Less frequent	
Sinus bradycardia		
Sinoatrial block		
Atrioventricular block		
Sinus tachycardia		
PVC		
Ventricular fibrillation		
Idioventricular rhythm		
Central Nervous System		
Confusion	Infrequent	Evaluate for impending toxicity.
Slurred speech	Rare	Evaluate for impending toxicity.
Coma	Rare	Support the patient. Reduce lithium SDC. Obtain chest X-ray, electrolytes.
Seizures	Rare	Support the patient. Reduce SDC with dialysis.
Ataxia	Rare	Evaluate for impending toxicity.
Dizziness	Rare	Tolerate or use slow-release preparation or administer with food to slow absorption and avoid peaks. Reduce lithium dosage.
Fine tremor/shakiness	4–45%	Wait. Slightly reduce lithium dosage. Reduce caffeine intake. Consider administration of a beta blocking agent. Coarse tremor is a sign of impending toxicity.
General weakness	33%	Wait; usually transient
Gastrointestinal		
Nausea	50%	Administer with food or use slow-release form. Avoid use of antiemetic which may mask toxicity. If occurs late in therapy, clinically evaluate for impending toxicity.
Vomiting	50%	Spread doses out throughout the day, change to slow-release product, or reduce lithium dose. Monitor electrolytes. If occurs late in therapy, clinically evaluate for impending toxicity
Diarrhea	20%	If on slow-release product consider change to a more rapidly and completely absorbed preparation.

TOXICITY	INCIDENCE	CLINICAL COMMENTS
Metallic taste in mouth or dry mouth	10–50%	Tolerate. Patient may use sugarless candy/fruit drinks. Consider dosage reduction
Renal		
Polyuria	50%	Consider reducing lithium dosage. Ensure adequate fluid intake. Closely monitor for signs of fluid and electrolyte imbalance.
Polydypsia	50%	Closely monitor for signs of fluid and electrolyte imbalance. Reduce lithium dose
Other		
Rash	Rare	Is usually self-limiting and resolves with continued lithium use. Consider discontinuing lithium until rash resolves. Lithium may be reinstituted
Reduced Sexual Ability	10%	Tolerate or reduce dosage
Weight gain	30%	Reduce caloric intake. Not fluid-related
Blurred vision	Rare	Consider dosage reduction
Swelling of extremities	Rare	Evaluate for sodium retention
Hypothyroidism Goiter	30% 4%	Check thyroid function studies to evaluate for hypothyroidism. Discontinue lithium as a last resort

DRUG INTERACTIONS

DRUGS CAUSING DECREASED LITHIUM CONCENTRATIONS	CLINICAL COMMENTS
Theophylline/aminophylline	−58%
Urea	−36%
Acetazolamide	−31%
Sodium bicarbonate	−27%
Spironolactone	−16%
DRUGS CAUSING INCREASED LITHIUM CONCENTRATIONS	
Indomethacin	+31%
Hydrochlorothiazide	+25%
Diclofenac	+23%
DRUGS AFFECTED BY LITHIUM	
Antipsychotic Drugs	
Chlorpromazine	Reduced chlorpromazine levels by 40%
Other phenothiazines (except thioridazine)	May mask the early signs of lithium intoxication, nausea and vomiting
Haloperidol	May mask the early signs of lithium intoxication, nausea and vomiting
Antihistamines	
Hydroxyzine	Enhanced cardiac toxicity
Antibiotics	
Tetracycline	Possible lithium toxicity at low lithium concentrations
Skeletal Muscle Relaxants	
Decamethonium	Potentiated or prolonged
Pancuronium bromide	Potentiated or prolonged
Succinylcholine	Potentiated or prolonged
Norepinephrine	Pressor effects may be decreased
Iodide preparations	Use may produce hypothyroidism
Other CNS depressants	Additive CNS depression

CLINICAL INTERPRETATION

- SDC data must be interpreted together with the patient's current clinical status, response, and pharmacokinetic considerations.

- Generally, the patient should be at steady-state (3–5 elimination half-lives) when sample is collected to ensure reliable interpretation of a SDC result. Time to peak SDC is usually 1–3h for immediate-release products. This will vary depending upon product formulation (i.e., sustained-release products will have a delayed time to peak). Time to achieve steady-state is approximately 3–7 days of chronic dosing.

- If only one measurement is going to be made, then a trough concentration provides the best guide for dosage adjustment.

Disease
- Renal dysfunction will ↑ SDC.
- States leading to dehydration will ↑ SDC.

Drugs
- Thiazide diuretics ↓ lithium renal secretion.
- Salt loading ↑ lithium renal excretion.
- Antipsychotic agents may ↑ neurologic toxicities due to lithium.

FACTORS AFFECTING EXCRETION

- Dehydrated patients retain lithium through renal mechanisms. However, water loading will not change lithium clearance significantly.

- Sodium deprivation causes potentially lethal toxicity as well as a compensatory lithium retention. The most dramatic example was the report of death in cardiac patients who used lithium chloride as a salt substitute.

- Lithium clearance in recumbent patients was 36% greater than when the same patients were ambulatory. Posture is known to affect the clearance of lithium. Slower nocturnal lithium clearance and circadian variations have been described.

- Causes of reduction in the clearance of lithium are; CHF, renal blood flow obstruction, volume contraction, hypertension, infection, renal toxins, and other disease states that reduce the GFR or renal function.

PHENOBARBITAL/ PRIMIDONE

CLINICAL PHARMACOKINETICS
SUMMARY TABLE

	Phenobarbital	Primidone (parent drug)
SERUM CONCENTRATIONS		
Minimum effective concentrations		
Seizures	15 µg/mL	5 µg/mL
Sedating ventilated neonates	60 µg/mL	not indicated
Potentially toxic concentrations		
Adults and children	>40 µg/mL	>12 µg/mL
Neonates	>60 µg/mL	>20 µg/mL
% BIOAVAILABILITY	90–100%	90–100%
TIME TO PEAK CONCENTRATION	1-3 h	1-3 h
TIME TO STEADY-STATE	3–4 wk	1–4 d
HALF-LIFE (T½)		
Adults	4d (53–140) h	8.0 (3.3–19) h
Children	1.5d (37–94) h	8.7 (4.5–11) h
Neonates	4d (43–404) h	Inadequate data
VOLUME OF DISTRIBUTION		
Adults and children	0.6 L/kg	0.65 (0.43–1.14) L/kg
Neonates	0.9 (0.7-1.2) L/kg	Inadequate data
CLEARANCE		
Total body clearance		
Adults	3.2 (2.1–4.1) mL/h/kg	Monotherapy: 30.9 mL/h/kg Combined therapy: 73.9 mL/h/kg
Children	8.2 (5.1–14.1) mL/h/kg	(32.7–102) mL/h/kg
Neonates	6.4 (2.7–17) mL/h/kg	
Geriatrics	2.4 (0.14–3.6) mL/h/kg	
Percent removed during hemodialysis (4 h)	30%	30%
% PROTEIN-BOUND	50%	≤20%
% EXCRETED RENALLY UNCHANGED		
Adults and children	20–40%	20–40%
Neonates	60–80%	Inadequate data
MAJOR ROUTE OF ELIMINATION	Hepatic: ~75% hepatic metabolism	Hepatic: 60–80% hepatic metabolism
ACTIVE METABOLITES	None	Phenobarbital: 3–5%, Phenylethylmalonamide (PEMA): 30–45%

THERAPEUTIC DRUG MONITORING

GENERAL GUIDELINES

- The patient should be at steady-state (2–5 elimination half-lives) or have received a loading dose to ensure reliable interpretation of the SDC result.

- Although phenobarbital is known to have hepatic enzyme induction properties, studies verify that the half-life during chronic therapy (mean ~100h) is longer than that upon initiation of therapy.

- Because of phenobarbital's long elimination half-life, sampling time is unimportant; however, when making comparative measurements, the sampling times relative to dosing should be consistent. For primidone, the trough level should be measured.

- Because primidone is partially metabolized to phenobarbital, serum trough concentrations of **both** drugs should be measured in patients receiving primidone.

SAMPLE COLLECTION

	SAMPLING TIME	CLINICAL COMMENTS
Initial Monitoring		
At onset of therapy	Phenobarbital: 2h after an "effective" IV loading dose to document the "effective" concentration	Repeat 3–4 wk after initiation of therapy after steady-state concentration has been attained
	Primidone: 3–4 wk after initiation	This allows concentrations of phenobarbital metabolites to reach steady-state
Resampling		
Following dose changes	3–4 wk after dose rate changes	Assures patient is at steady state
Following addition or discontinuation of known enzyme-inducer	3–4 wk after concomitant therapy change	Assures patient is at steady state
Evidence of toxicity or overdose	Immediately for both phenobarbital and primidone	Document toxicity
Loss of seizure control	Immediately for both phenobarbital and primidone	To reference SDC
Pregnancy	Frequently during pregnancy and for 8 wk after delivery	Monitor SDC's closely due to physiologic changes

CLINICAL MONITORING PARAMETERS

- ♦ Hepatic Function
- ♦ Renal Function
- ♦ Hematopoietic Function

THERAPEUTICS

USUAL DOSING PARAMETERS

DRUG	PATIENT GROUP	INITIAL DOSE	DAILY MAINTENANCE	APPROXIMATE T½ NORMAL RENAL FUNCTION
Phenobarbital	Adults & children >10–15 yr	10–30 mg/kg	1.5–2.0 mg/kg/d	~4 d
	Children <10 yr	15–40 mg/kg Divided dose q 12–24 h	3–4.5 mg/kg/d	~2 d
	Neonates	15–45 mg/kg	5 mg/kg/d (2.5 mg/kg/d if seizures due to neonatal or perinatal asphyxia)	~4 d
Primidone	Adults & children	See below	10–25 mg/kg/d Divided dose q 6–8 h	~8 h
	Neonates	See below	12–20 mg/kg/d	Variable Divided dose q 6–8 h

CLINICAL COMMENTS

♦ PHENOBARBITAL Loading dose may be given by oral, IM, or IV route. Only the IV routes provide rapid peak concentration consistently. May give entire initial dose or divide into 2–3 smaller doses over several hours. IV doses should not be administered faster than 50–100 mg/min in adults.

Dosage Form	Form	% Active Drug	Strengths
Tablets	Free acid	100%	100 mg, 65 mg, 30 mg, 15 mg
Elixir	Free acid	100%	20 mg/5 mL
Injectable	Sodium salt	91%	30 mg/mL, 60 mg/mL, 130 mg/mL

♦ PRIMIDONE Loading doses are not advised. An initial dose of 50–125 mg in adults should be given. Dose rates should be increased by 50–125 mg increments every 2–4 d until the desired maintenance dose is achieved. Higher maintenance doses may be necessary for patients taking phenytoin or carbamazepine concurrently.

Dosage Form	Form	% Active Drug	Strengths
Tablets	Free acid	100%	50 mg, 250 mg
Suspension	Free acid	100%	250 mg/5 mL

COMMON TOXICITIES AND ADVERSE REACTIONS

TOXICITY	INCIDENCE	CLINICAL COMMENTS
Cardiac/Vascular Hypotension	Rare	Related to rapid IV Phenobarbital infusion, i.e., a rate > 50–100 mg/min in adults
Hypersensitivity		
Skin rashes	1–3%	Most rashes disappear over several days after stopping drug
Stevens-Johnson syndrome	≤1–3%	
Idiosyncratic Reactions		
Frozen shoulder syndrome	<6%	Middle-aged patients usually affected
Low folic acid	27–91%	Mainly seen when polypharmacy used; anemia rare
Neonatal bleeding	Uncommon	Prevented by giving vitamin K at delivery
Osteomalacia	Uncommon	Symptoms rare although biochemical evidence is more common
Porphyria	>50%	May precipitate acute attack in patients with acute intermittent porphyria
Shoulder-hand syndrome	Rare	Most common if primidone dose >1000 mg
Neurosensory Agitation Depression Drowsiness Fatigue Sedation	>50%	Higher incidence when therapy initiated, tolerance develops in most patients
Impaired higher cortical function		Occurs in most patients beginning at lower therapeutic concentrations
Hyperactivity (children only)	40%	Seen primarily in children, uncommon in elderly patients
Teratogenesis	Rare	Reports with monotherapy appear to occur when phenobarbital plasma concentration ≥70 μg/mL
Withdrawal symptoms Anxiety Confusion Diaphoresis Emotional lability Insomnia Seizures Tremors	>50% if drug abruptly discontinued	Some symptoms expected in most patients and may last days to several weeks; should use gradual tapering to discontinue drugs after chronic therapy

DRUG INTERACTIONS

DRUG	MECHANISM	CLINICAL COMMENTS
Drugs That Affect Phenobarbital Serum Concentrations		
Chloramphenicol Cimetidine Phenytoin Valproic acid	Enzyme inhibition	The phenobarbital dosage may need to be ↓ if these drugs are given concurrently. SDC monitoring is necessary after starting or stopping therapy.
Ethanol	Enzyme induction	Chronic ethanol use may ↑ phenobarbital requirements.
Drugs That Affect Primidone Serum Concentrations		
Isoniazid (INH)	Enzyme inhibition	Primidone SDC ↑ with concurrent ↓ in phenobarbital and PEMA concentrations. Monitor SDC closely.
Phenytoin Carbamazepine	Enzyme induction	Primidone SDC are ↓, phenobarbital SDC are ↑. Higher dosage and shorter dosing intervals may be required.
Valproic acid	Enzyme inhibition	May cause ↑ in both phenobarbital and primidone concentrations, requiring close monitoring of SDC.
Primidone/Phenobarbital Effects on Other Drugs		
Enzyme Induction Carbamazepine Corticosteroids Chlorpromazine Doxycycline Oral contraceptives Quinidine Tricyclic antidepressants Warfarin	Altered metabolism	Metabolism of these drugs is ↑ requiring higher dose rates to get adequate response.
Furosemide	Unknown	↓ diuresis
Phenytoin	Altered Metabolism	Concurrent use may either ↑ phenytoin SDC through competitive inhibition or parahydroxylation, or ↓ phenytoin SDC through enzyme induction. Close monitoring of phenytoin concentration is necessary.

CLINICAL INTERPRETATION

Data must be interpreted together with the patient's current clinical status, response, and pharmacokinetic considerations.

- For primidone, the relationship between SDC and seizure control is complicated by its active metabolite, phenobarbital.

Concomitant Drug Therapy

- Clonazepam and valproic acid may increase the SDC of phenobarbital and/or primidone. Phenytoin can increase the concentration of phenobarbital by as much as 40%.

Age

- Adults have longer elimination half-lives than children.

Disease

- No definitive statements can be made on exactly to what degree renal, cardiac, or hepatic dysfunction will affect the disposition of these drugs. However, decreased phenobarbital metabolism is expected in patients with impaired hepatic function, and renal clearance is probably affected in patients with impaired renal function. These patients should be carefully monitored.

PHENYTOIN

CLINICAL PHARMACOKINETICS
SUMMARY TABLE

SERUM CONCENTRATIONS		
Minimum effective concentration		10 µg/mL
Potentially toxic concentration		>20 µg/mL
Neonate to 3-mo-old therapeutic range		6–14 µg/mL
% BIOAVAILABILITY		85–95%
TIME TO PEAK CONCENTRATION		1.5–48 h depending on dosage form
Dilantin Kapseals		3 h
TIME TO STEADY-STATE		7–10 d
HALF-LIFE (T½)	Pre-term neonate	3 d ± 65 h
	Term neonate <1 wk	1 d ± 12 h
	Infants 2 wk to 3 mo	8h ±
	>3 mo	8h ±
	Children	8h ±
	Adults	20–40 h
	Pregnancy	Decreased
VOLUME OF DISTRIBUTION	Pre-term neonate	0.5 L/kg
	Term neonate	0.8 L/kg
	Adult	0.7 L/kg
CLEARANCE		
Total body clearance		22 mL/h/kg ± 0.2 mL/h/kg
Michaelis constant (K_m)		4 µg/mL (mean) 1–15 µg/mL (range)
Maximum rate of metabolism (V_{max})		7 mg/kg/d (mean) 1.4–14 mg/kg/d (range)
Percent removed from the body during hemodialysis (6h)		4%
% PROTEIN-BOUND	Adults	90%
	Infants (0–12 wk)	65%
% EXCRETED RENALLY UNCHANGED		<5%
MAJOR ROUTE OF ELIMINATION	Hepatic	>95%
ACTIVE METABOLITES		None

THERAPEUTIC DRUG MONITORING

GENERAL GUIDELINES

- Generally, the patient should have received the drug for at least 3–5 elimination half-lives before the sample is collected to ensure reliable interpretation of the SDC.

- Trough levels should be monitored to measure the minimum SDC during the dosing interval. In children, however, serum phenytoin concentration may fluctuate substantially during a dosing interval, necessitating serial SDC for complete characterization.

- Trough concentrations should be measured 1 wk after initiating therapy and then again 3–5 wk later.

- Peak concentration may be useful in confirming toxicity. IV peak will occur within 2–4 h after IV loading dose.

SAMPLE COLLECTION

	WHEN TO SAMPLE	CLINICAL COMMENTS
Initial Monitoring		
At onset of therapy	2 wk–1 mo after initiation	Immediately before next oral dose. Generally, 3–5 elimination half-lives before the sample is collected. If loading dose is used, steady-state will be achieved earlier
Resampling Guidelines		
Following dose changes	After 2 wk–1 mo	To establish reference point for future dosage adjustments
Loss of seizure control, when there are signs of toxicity, or following an overdose	Immediately	To determine possible causes (e.g., poor compliance, rapid metabolism toxicity, refractiveness to treatment)
Possible drug interactions	2 wk–1 mo following addition or discontinuation of the interacting drug	Potentially serious interactions should be assessed more quickly even though SDC may not be at steady-state.
Development of illnesses that may alter phenytoin metabolism	Immediately	Altered phenytoin disposition with hepatic or renal disease
During pregnancy	Frequently during and after	Monitor 2–4 wk after delivery to gauge changing phenytoin dose requirements
Following changes in oral dosage formulation	2 wk–1 mo after the change	Significant bioavailability change occurs with some formulations. Avoid generics unless their quality is well documented
Suspicion of laboratory error	Immediately	An alternative method may be appropriate in some cases

CLINICAL MONITORING PARAMETERS

- ♦ Serum calcium
- ♦ CBC
- ♦ Hepatic function
- ♦ Periodic dental examination
- ♦ Physical examination for lymph node enlargement

THERAPEUTICS

USUAL DOSING PARAMETERS

PATIENT GROUP	LOADING OR INITIAL DOSE (mg/kg)	MAINTENANCE DOSE RATE (mg/kg/d)	DOSING INTERVAL
Newborns and infants <3 mo	15–20	3–5	8 h
Children 6 mo–6 yr	10–15	5–15	8–12 h
Adults	13–15	5–7	8–24 h
Pregnancy	13–15	5–15	8–24 h

CLINICAL COMMENTS

- **Children:**
  In children, some experts recommend 5–15 mg/kg/d for a maintenance dose. The higher dose is required secondary to higher body clearances. Newborns absorb phenytoin poorly; IV therapy is recommended. Higher dose rate required because of higher body clearance. Higher dose rates and shorter intervals may be necessary in polytherapy.

- **During Pregnancy:**
  Dose rate adjustments should be individualized and increases made only if there is loss of seizure control.

- **Loading Doses:**
  If oral, the loading dose should be given in 3 divided doses over a 4h period; if IV, loading dose should be infused slowly at a rate not exceeding 50 mg/min. Maintenance therapy should be initiated within 12h following the loading dose.

PRODUCT FORMULATIONS CAN VARY SIGNIFICANTLY

DRUG	CLINICAL COMMENTS
Sodium phenytoin injectable (50 mg/mL)	Adjusted pH to 12, contains propylene glycol 40% and alcohol 10%; administer IV at a rate no faster than 50 mg/min; not recommended for IM administration due to erratic absorption; do not mix with glucose solutions; 92% phenytoin (46 mg/mL)
Sodium phenytoin capsules (30 mg, 100 mg)	Most widely used preparation; 92% phenytoin (28 mg, 92 mg)
Phenytoin tablet (50 mg)	Chewable; convenient for pediatric use; 100% phenytoin
Phenytoin suspension (30 mg/5 mL, 125 mg/5 mL)	Shake well, may concentrate in the bottom; use caution in making precise measurements (teaspoon size variable); do not mix pediatric and adult strengths; may be used in patients who absorb the capsules poorly; 100% phenytoin

COMMON TOXICITIES AND ADVERSE REACTIONS

TOXICITY	INCIDENCE	CLINICAL COMMENTS
Dose-related Behavioral changes Coma Drowsiness Higher cortical dysfunction Incoordination Nystagmus Visual blurring	15–38%	Higher incidence at initiation of therapy; nystagmus usually earliest sign; usual progression of nystagmus, ataxia, higher cortical dysfunction; in some patients toxic symptoms may be apparent at levels below the usual therapeutic range.
Pharmacologic Toxicities		
Acne Hirsutism, coarse facial features	5–10%	Generally mild; usually more disturbing to women; rarely requires discontinuation of therapy
Folic acid deficiency	~5%	Folic acid deficiency and a megaloblastic anemia have been reported in association with phenytoin. A prospective study confirmed the reduction in serum and red cell folic acid but detected no evidence of anemia or alteration of other hematologic parameters. It appears that complicating factors, such as diet, may contribute to the megaloblastic anemia seen with phenytoin therapy
Gingival hyperplasia	30–50%	May lead to malocclusion; good oral hygiene recommended; rarely requires discontinuation of therapy
Cerebellar degeneration	Rare	Repeated seizures may be contributory; cellular syndrome may develop
Hypothyroidism	Rare	Biochemical evidence common, but symptoms are rare
Immunologic disturbances	20–60%	Alterations of various cellular and/or humoral immune responses have been described. Reduced IgA is most commonly seen, but changes in IgM and IgG have also been reported.
Osteomalacia	Uncommon	Symptoms uncommon; bio-chemical evidence is common; serum calcium and alkaline phosphatase should be monitored
Peripheral neuropathy	Rare	Generally subclinical; may result in depressed deep tendon reflexes
Hypersensitivity		
Skin rashes	1–10%	The morbilliform rash is the most common and is usually self-limited. If severe, may require discontinuation of therapy; generally occurs within first few weeks of therapy

TOXICITY	INCIDENCE	CLINICAL COMMENTS
Exfoliative dermatitis	Rare	
Erythema multiforme	Rare	
Stevens-Johnson syndrome	Rare	
Pseudolymphoma	Rare	
Idiosyncratic reactions		
Anemia	Rare	Although anemia is rare, megaloblastic changes and macrocytosis are common
Aplastic anemia	Rare	
Erythroid hyperplasia	Rare	
Hepatitis	Rare	May occur with pseudolymphoma; rash generally present; eosinophilia is common; hepatic function should be monitored regularly at intervals. Fatal hepatic necrosis can occur
Leukopenia	Rare	Hematologic parameters should be monitored at intervals
Lupus-like reaction	Rare	
Teratogenicity	6–10%	Two- to three-fold increase; most commonly observed malformations include cleft lip and palate and cardiac septal defects; fetal hydantoin syndrome is rare; specific risk to an individual patient is unknown; during pregnancy, should maintain plasma levels at lowest that will maintain seizure control
Thrombocytopenia	Rare	

DRUG INTERACTIONS

DRUG	MECHANISM	CLINICAL COMMENTS
Drugs That Alter Phenytoin SDC		
Bioavailability		
Antacids	Reduced extent of absorption	Phenytoin SDC ↓
Hepatic Metabolism		
Bishydroxycoumarin Chloramphenicol Cimetidine Disulfiram Isoniazid Methsuximide Phenylbutazone Propoxyphene Sulfonamides	Enzyme inhibition	Phenytoin SDC ↑; lower daily doses and longer dosing intervals may be required; SDC monitoring is important after initiation of therapy with these drugs and after their discontinuation
Carbamazepine Ethanol Phenobarbital	Enzyme induction	Phenytoin SDC ↓; higher daily doses and shorter dosing intervals may be required
Effects on Protein Binding		
Salicylates	Phenytoin displacement from serum proteins	Total phenytoin SDC may be lower, but no change in dosing should be necessary
Phenylbutazone Valproic Acid	Phenytoin displacement from serum proteins and enzyme inhibition	Phenytoin SDC may be reduced because of higher unbound fractions; unbound SDC may be higher because of enzyme inhibition. A reduction in daily dosage of phenytoin may be necessary

DRUG	MECHANISM	CLINICAL COMMENTS
Phenytoin's Effects on Other Drugs		
Bishydroxycoumarin	Enzyme induction, protein binding displacement	Decreased anticoagulation effect; if phenytoin is discontinued, hemorrhagic complications may result
Carbamazepine	Enzyme induction	↓ carbamazepine SDC result; a higher daily dose and more frequent administration of carbamazepine may be necessary
Oral contraceptives	Increased clearance	Reduced efficacy is possible; higher incidence of withdrawal bleeding
Primidone	Enzyme induction	↑ metabolism of primidone resulting in ↑ SDC of derived phenobarbital
Steroids	Increased clearance	Higher doses of steroids may be required
Acetaminophen Doxycycline Folic acid Pyridoxine Quinidine Vitamin D	Increased clearance	Potential reduction in drug efficacy; higher doses may be required

CLINICAL INTERPRETATION

Phenytoin SDC must be interpreted in conjunction with the patient's current clinical status, seizure history, and pharmacokinetic parameters. The therapeutic range is usually 10–20 μg/mL for adults/children and 6–14 μg/mL for neonates/pre-term to 12 weeks. There are a number of factors that affect phenytoin SDC and interpretations. Some of these important factors are:

Altered Protein Binding

- Renal failure: accumulation of 5-(hydroxphenyl)-5-phenylhydantoin (HPPH) metabolite or a binding inhibitor can displace phenytoin from albumin binding sites.
- Reduced albumin concentration: hypoalbuminemia may be present in liver or renal disease, resulting in more unbound phenytoin.
- Age: infants 0–12 wk old have reduced phenytoin protein binding.
- Unbound Drug: May increase concentration of "unbound" drug.
- Concomitant drug therapy: acidic drugs can displace phenytoin from its binding sites (e.g., salicylates, valproic acid, phenylbutazone, sulfonylureas).
- Metabolic waste products: Elevated levels of metabolic waste products (e.g., bilirubin and urea) can displace phenytoin from albumin binding sites.

Factors That May Decrease Phenytoin SDC

- Acute hepatitis
- Age (infants 0–12 wk); ability to metabolize phenytoin increases to rates exceeding those found in adults during first 2 wk of life
- Alcohol
- Mononucleosis
- Pregnancy (increased plasma clearance)
- Renal disease (increased hepatic metabolism)

Factors That May Increase Phenytoin SDC

- Chronic liver disease (decreased metabolism)
- Concomitant drug therapy: barbiturates (particularly high concentrations), carbamazepine, chloramphenicol, disulfiram, isoniazid, dicumarol
- Hepatic immaturity (pre-term infants)

PROCAINAMIDE/ NAPA

CLINICAL PHARMACOKINETICS
SUMMARY TABLE

SERUM CONCENTRATIONS		
Minimum effective concentrations	Procainamide	4 μg/mL
	Sum of procainamide and NAPA	10 μg/mL
Potentially toxic concentrations	Procainamide	>10 μg/mL
	Sum of procainamide and NAPA	>30 μg/mL
% BIOAVAILABILITY		83% ± 16% (variable)
TIME TO PEAK CONCENTRATION	IV	15–30 min after infusion
	PO	75 min (range: 1–4 h)
	PO (extended-release product)	>2 h
TIME TO STEADY-STATE	Normal renal function	~1 d
	↓ renal function	~2–3 d
HALF-LIFE (T½)	Adults	3.3 h ± 0.64 h
	Children	1.7 h ± 0.1 h
VOLUME OF DISTRIBUTION		
Central compartment		
Adults		0.67 ± 0.13 L/kg
Children		Inadequate data
At steady-state		
Adults		2.0 ± 0.42 L/kg
CLEARANCE		
Total body clearance		
Adults		8.6 ± 1.9 mL/min/kg
Children		19.4 ± 2.0 mL/min/kg
Hemodialysis clearance		
Adults	Varies with dialysis machine; similar for NAPA	68 mL/min
Children		Inadequate data
% PROTEIN-BOUND		15%
% EXCRETED RENALLY UNCHANGED		52% ± 11%
MAJOR ROUTE OF ELIMINATION	Renal excretion and hepatic metabolism	
ACTIVE METABOLITES	NAPA (acecanide)	20–50% metabolized to NAPA

THERAPEUTIC DRUG MONITORING

GENERAL GUIDELINES

Some patients taking procainamide absorb the drug slowly; therefore, their procainamide SDC may be higher at the end of the dosing interval. Decisions regarding procainamide dosing based on the results of a single SDC may be inappropriate. Ideally, 3 blood samples should be collected during a steady-state dosing interval: 1 when the dose is given and the others at equally spaced intervals. If only 2 samples are obtained, then they should be collected at the end of the dosing interval and 2h following the dose. Because the procainamide metabolite NAPA is pharmacologically active, SDC of both should be obtained to optimize drug therapy.

Indications for Measuring Serum Procainamide Concentrations

♦ Poor predictability of dose-response relationship	Procainamide pharmacokinetics may vary greatly among patients
Active metabolite (NAPA)	NAPA SDC cannot be predicted accurately; NAPA must be calculated in overall therapeutic level; combined therapeutic range from 10–30 μg/mL
♦ Determine appropriate oral dose after IV therapy	
♦ Assess adequacy of therapy	Subtherapeutic SDC
♦ Changes in patient's underlying status may alter pharmacokinetics and SDC	Renal dysfunction Fast acetylators (>120 mL/min) Slow acetylators (<80 mL/min) (heightened SLE risk if slow)
♦ Assess acetylator phenotype (procainamide and NAPA levels)	

SAMPLE COLLECTION

	WHEN TO SAMPLE
Oral Dosing Draw blood samples only when steady-state is achieved	Usually, 2 full days; if loading dose given, steady-state will occur sooner; in cases of renal dysfunction, time to steady-state will be prolonged
Timing of Samples 3 samples (ideal) When dose is administered Middle of dosing interval End of dosing interval 2 samples End of dosing interval 2h after dose is administered	Peak: ~75min after an oral dose of prompt release products, e.g. Pronestyl. However peak concentrations may not occur until 2–4 h or more following an oral dose of Pronestyl in some patients and in all patients receiving sustained release products.
Single sample	Trough: Immediately before next oral dose
Intravenous Dosing 2–infusion technique	Immediately after IV loading infusion; 2h after start of IV maintenance infusion; 6–12 h after start of IV maintenance infusion; 24h after start of IV maintenance therapy

NOTE: Neither sample should exceed 15 μg/mL
Loading infusion level should be higher than maintenance infusion level

CLINICAL MONITORING PARAMETERS

- Antinuclear antibody tests (to detect SLE)
- BP (during IV administration)
- Cardiac function
- CBC

THERAPEUTICS

USUAL DOSING PARAMETERS

PATIENT GROUP	INITIAL DOSE	DAILY MAINTENANCE	APPROXIMATE T½ NORMAL RENAL FUNCTION
Pediatrics			
Oral Dosing		40–60 mg/kg/d divided q 4–6 h	~1.7h
IV Dosing		2 mg/kg/dose (max dose 100 mg) given slowly and repeated q 10–30 min; max daily dose 1–2 g	
Adult			
IV Dosing			
No renal impairment and no evidence of severe CHF	17 mg/kg over 1 h	2.8–3.0 mg/kg/h	~3.3h
Moderate renal impairment (BUN 25–40 mg/100 mL)	17 mg/kg over 1 h	2.0 mg/kg/h	(↑)
Severe renal impairment (BUN >40 mg/100 mL), pulmonary edema, or cardiogenic shock	14 mg/kg over 1 h	1.0 mg/kg/h	(↑)
Oral Dosing	2x maintenance dose	Same as IV (above); dosing interval approximates drug half-life	~3.3h
Oral Dosing After Lidocaine Infusion	2x procainamide oral maintenance dose	Decrease lidocaine maintenance infusion by 25% when second procainamide dose is given Repeat until lidocaine infusion is discontinued at end of 4th procainamide (PA) dosage interval	

CLINICAL COMMENTS

- Pediatric doses are based on limited data.
- Maximum PO daily dose in children = 2–4 g, maximum IV daily dose in children = 1–2 g.
- Adjust maintenance dose for reduced renal and cardiac output
- Any alteration in PA dosage should be guided by SDC determinations and patient response.
- Some patients may fail to respond to PA SDC in the range of 10–15 μg/mL. Inadequate response at these levels should indicate consideration of alternate therapy.
- When given as an IV bolus or by rapid IV infusion, PA can cause excessive slowing of the heart rate and dangerous hypotension.

COMMON TOXICITIES AND ADVERSE REACTIONS

TOXICITY	INCIDENCE	CLINICAL COMMENTS
Arrhythmias	Uncommon	Usually associated with excessive rate of administration or concentration of PA + NAPA > 25–30 μg/mL
Bradycardia	Common	Usually not clinically significant
Dizziness, light-headedness	Uncommon	
Drug-induced SLE	Common	Usually reversible by PA discontinuation; may occur in 30% of patients receiving chronic therapy
Hypotension	Common	Usually not clinically significant
Mental confusion, mental depression, hallucinations	Rare	
Myocardial depression	Uncommon	Patients with significantly impaired myocardial function at increased risk
Nausea, vomiting, diarrhea, anorexia	Common	May disappear with continued use; rarely seen when procainamide plus NAPA SDC is < 30 μg/mL
Prolongation of ECG intervals	Common	Usually not clinically significant

DRUG INTERACTIONS

DRUG	MECHANISM	CLINICAL COMMENTS
Amiodarone	Unknown	Variable onset and magnitude of increased procainamide SDC
Antiarrhythmics		May produce additive effects
Cholinergics	Cholinergic-blocking action	Particularly important in persons with myasthenia gravis, prolonged or enhanced effects of cholinergic agent
Cimetidine	Decreased renal clearance	Effect can be clinically significant; monitor PA SDC when cimetidine is started or stopped
Ethanol	Increased acetylation	Limited information available, but appears to be clinically significant

CLINICAL INTERPRETATION

Factors Affecting Procainamide Serum Concentrations

FACTOR	CLINICAL COMMENTS
♦ Acetylator phenotype	Higher concentrations of NAPA in fast acetylators.
♦ Age	↓ in PA renal clearance may be greater than age-related ↓ in GFR
♦ Cardiogenic shock	↓ clearance results in ↑ SDC
♦ Congestive heart failure	Limited data available, but dose rate should probably be ↓ in patients with moderate to severe CHF
♦ Decreased PA bioavailability in some patients	May result in inadequate response in spite of "appropriate" dosing
♦ Drug interactions	Effect dependent on interacting drug
♦ Hemodialysis	Replacement doses may be necessary
♦ Hepatic disease	Limited data available; presence of significant hepatic disease may warrant ↓ in dose
♦ Intrapatient variability in relative bioavailability of PA from sustained-release and immediate-release preparations	Monitor patient at C_{ss} after change in dose or dosing interval
♦ Pulmonary edema	↓ clearance causes ↑ SDC
♦ Renal impairment	↓ renal function results in ↓ clearance of both PA and NAPA

QUINIDINE

CLINICAL PHARMACOKINETICS
SUMMARY TABLE

SERUM CONCENTRATIONS		
Minimum effective concentration		2.3 μg/mL
Potentially toxic concentration		> 5 μg/mL
% BIOAVAILABILITY	PO	70–80%
	IM	Incomplete absorption
TIME TO PEAK CONCENTRATION	Sulfate (rapid-release)	1–2 h
	Gluconate (slow- or sustained-released)	4–6 h
TIME TO STEADY-STATE	Chronic dosing	30–35 h
HALF-LIFE (T½)*	Adults	6–7 h (range: 1.6–16 h)
	Pediatrics (limited data)	~6 h
VOLUME OF DISTRIBUTION		~3.0 L/kg
CLEARANCE		
Total body clearance		4.70 mL/min/kg
% excreted unchanged in urine		pH dependent
% metabolized by the liver		60% (normals)
% removed by dialysis		Inadequate data
Renal clearance		0.93 mL/min/kg
% PROTEIN-BOUND		80–90%
% EXCRETED RENALLY UNCHANGED		10–30%; renal excretion is pH dependent
MAJOR ROUTE OF ELIMINATION	Hepatic	
ACTIVE METABOLITES	3-hydroxyquinidine, quinidine-N-oxide, quinidine 10, 11-dihydrodiol	Some of these metabolites may have cardioactivity and may interfere with some assay methodologies

NOTE: The T½ may be prolonged in patients with cirrhosis or end-stage hepatic disease and in patients with severe heart failure.

THERAPEUTIC DRUG MONITORING

GENERAL GUIDELINES

♦ Generally, the patient should be at steady-state (3–5 elimination half-lives) when a sample is collected to ensure reliable interpretation of an SDC.

Indications For Measuring Serum Quinidine Concentrations

Toxicity is suspected	Drug-drug interactions
Patient compliance	Change in product formulation
Patient-specific kinetic variability	Change in dose or dosing schedule
Drug-disease interactions	

Normal Time To Steady-state	Adults: 30–35 h May be prolonged in patients with severe heart failure or end-stage liver disease

SAMPLE COLLECTION

♦ Since quinidine absorption characteristics may vary widely among patients, and at times within the same patient, a trough concentration generally provides the most reliable index of the quinidine SDC. In general these concentrations should be determined at steady-state to ensure reliable interpretation.

WHEN TO SAMPLE	Peak	Quinidine sulfate[1]: ~1h after oral dose Quinidex[2] Extentabs: 2–3 h after oral dose Quinidine gluconate: ~5h after oral dose
	Trough	Immediately before next oral dose

♦ Definition of minimum effective SDC, potentially toxic SDC, and the therapeutic range for quinidine may depend on the assay method used. Clinicians requesting quinidine levels should ask that the analytical method be specified (see page 118).

CLINICAL MONITORING PARAMETERS

- CBC
- Hepatic Function
- Renal Function
- ECG
- Serum Potassium

THERAPEUTICS

USUAL DOSING PARAMETERS

PATIENT GROUP	INITIAL DOSE	DAILY MAINTENANCE	APPROXIMATE T½ NORMAL RENAL FUNCTION
Pediatric	2 mg/kg/dose (test dose)	5–30 mg/kg/d of **sulfate**; 3–6 mg/kg/ dose q 2–3 h; **gluconate**; 2–10 mg/kg/dose repeated q 3–6 h prn	~6h Pediatric dosing is based on limited data
Adult	400–800 mg PO. IV dose of **quinidine gluconate** 0.2–0.3 mg/kg slowly over 25–45 min	800–2400 mg/d **sulfate salt**; 660–2970 mg/d **gluconate salt**; given in divided doses	6–7 h (range: 1.6–16 h)

CLINICAL COMMENTS

- Some available assays for quinidine are nonspecific for parent drug.
- Because of the potential for hypersensitivity reaction, a test dose is recommended.
- When quinidine is added to digoxin therapy, the digoxin dose may need to be reduced and SDC monitored.
- Sustained release products facilitate enhanced patient compliance.

COMMON TOXICITIES AND ADVERSE REACTIONS

Side effects and/or toxicity may occur in as many as 30% of the patients receiving quinidine. It is difficult to determine the precise incidence of side effects in the general population.

TOXICITY	INCIDENCE	CLINICAL COMMENTS
♦ **Common Side Effects or Pharmacologic Toxicities**		
Gastrointestinal tract Loss of appetite Diarrhea Nausea Vomiting Abdominal pain or cramping Bitter taste	~50%	Appear to be dose-dependent in most patients; tolerance may develop, but these effects are the most common cause for discontinuing quinidine
Cardiovascular Bradycardia Hypotension Slow intraventricular conduction Re-entrant arrhythmias PVCs Ventricular tachycardia AV block Syncope	~18%	Patients with borderline cardiac compensation may be more susceptible to quinidine's depressant effects
♦ **Less Common or Rare Side Effects or Toxicities**		
Cinchonism	~7%	A constellation of disturbances (e.g., tinnitus, light-headedness, giddiness)
Hypersensitivity Reactions Drug fever Pulmonary distress (asthma, respiratory depression) Anaphylactic shock Hepatitis Rashes (exfoliative dermatitis, urticaria, scarlatiniform eruptions, morbilliform)	~7%	Drug fever may occur in as many as 12% of the patients receiving guideline doses

TOXICITY	INCIDENCE	CLINICAL COMMENTS
Severe erythrodermic exacerbations of psoriasis Lichenoid reactions Contact dermatitis Cutaneous lupus erythematosus		Rashes occur in about 7% of patients
Hematologic Reactions Thrombocytopenia Eosinophilia Hemolytic anemia Red cell antigen G-6-PD Agranulocytosis	1%	
Teratogenicity Eighth cranial nerve damage	Rare	The true incidence is unknown

DRUG INTERACTIONS

DRUG	MECHANISM	CLINICAL COMMENTS
Acetazolamide	↑ tubular reabsorption	↑ serum quinidine
Antacids	↑ tubular reabsorption	↑ serum quinidine
Anticoagulants	Additive hypoprothrombinemic effects	↑ risk of bleeding
Barbiturates	Enhanced metabolism	↓ serum quinidine
Cimetidine	Inhibits hepatic metabolism	↑ serum quinidine
Digitalis glycosides	Reduction of clearance	↑ serum glycosides
Neuromuscular blocking agents	Potentiates both non-depolarizing and depolarizing muscle relaxants	↑ neuromuscular blocking effect
Phenothiazines	Additive antiarrhythmic activity	Prolonged QT interval
Phenytoin	Enhanced metabolism	↓ serum quinidine
Rifampin	Enhanced metabolism	↓ serum quinidine
Sodium bicarbonate	↑ tubular reabsorption	↑ serum quinidine

CLINICAL INTERPRETATION

♦ There are a number of factors that can significantly affect the SDC of quinidine and/or the SDC-response relationship.

Factor	Effect
Severe heart failure (↓ clearance)	↑ SDC
Severely impaired hepatic function (e.g., end-stage liver disease; ↓ clearance)	↑ SDC
Concomitant drug therapy: urinary alkalizers (e.g., acetazolamide, antacids, sodium bicarbonate)	↑ SDC
Age (reduced clearance in elderly patients)	↑ SDC
Concomitant drug therapy: enzyme-inducing drugs (e.g., phenytoin)	↓ SDC
Collection tubes	↓ SDC
Hypokalemia	↑ pharmacologic effect
Altered protein binding (e.g., hypoalbuminemia)	↑ free drug which ↑ effect

♦ Many routinely available assays for quinidine are generally non-specific. More specific assays such as the chromatographic ones (gas, liquid, or thin-layer) will have a therapeutic range lower than usual. The double-extraction fluorometric assay measures quinidine, dihydroquinidine, and various amounts of metabolites; the quinidine-specific assays usually measure either quinidine or quinidine plus dihydroquinidine. Dihydroquinidine is a pharmacologically active constituent of quinidine preparations. Dihydroquinidine SDC are ~5-10% of the total quinidine SDC.

♦ Decreased renal function results in accumulation of metabolites in plasma, which may interfere with non-specific assays.

♦ When quinidine is added to digoxin therapy, the digoxin dose may need to be reduced and SDC monitored.

♦ Conflicting evidence exists about the effects of altered renal function and congestive heart failure on quinidine disposition.

♦ The major metabolites (3s)-3-hydroxyquinidine and 2-oxoquinidinone possess antiarrhythmic activity in animals; clinical relevance in man remains to be determined.

THEOPHYLLINE

CLINICAL PHARMACOKINETICS
SUMMARY TABLE

SERUM CONCENTRATIONS		
Minimum effective concentrations	Asthma	10 μg/mL
	Neonatal apnea	5 μg/mL
Potentially toxic concentrations	Generally minor adverse effects	>20–35 μg/mL
	Potential for cardiac arrhythmias, seizures, and death	> 35 μg/mL
% BIOAVAILABILITY	Oral	100%
	Rectal solutions	90%
	Rectal suppositories	Erratic
TIME TO PEAK CONCENTRATION	Depends on product formulation; average sustained-release product	~4 h
TIME TO STEADY-STATE		
Adults		~2 d
Pediatrics	Children	~1–2 d
	Premature neonates	~6 d
	Newborns	~5 d
	Infants	~1–5 d
HALF-LIFE (T½)		
Adults	Nonsmokers	~8.7 h
	Smokers	~4.4 h
	Patients with cardiac decomposition or hepatic cirrhosis	~20–30 h
Children	1–9 yr old	~3.7 h; half-life ↑ with age beyond 9 yr to adult
Neonates and infants	Prematures	~30 h
	Normal newborns	~24 h
	Infants beyond neonatal period	Gradually decreases from newborn level to childhood level by 1 yr of age
VOLUME OF DISTRIBUTION	Higher in neonates and patients with hepatic failure	0.5 L/kg (range: 0.3–0.7 L/kg)
CLEARANCE		
Adults	Healthy, non-smoking	0.65 mL/kg/min
Pediatrics	Newborns (premature)	0.29 mL/kg/min
	Younger children (1–4 yr)	1.4 mL/kg/min
	Older children (4–17 yr)	1.7 mL/kg/min
% PROTEIN-BOUND		
Adults		~60%
Neonates, and adults with liver cirrhosis		~36%

% EXCRETED RENALLY UNCHANGED		
Adults and children		7–13%
Term infants and premature newborns		35–50%
MAJOR ROUTE OF ELIMINATION	Hepatic metabolism with renal excretion of metabolites	
ACTIVE METABOLITES	3–methylxanthine has some activity, but quantities are too small to exert a pharmacologic effect	In neonates, 10% of theophylline is converted to caffeine. Another 4% is converted to theobromine.

THERAPEUTIC DRUG MONITORING

GENERAL GUIDELINES

- The therapeutic range for theophylline is narrow; risks of adverse reactions and potentially serious toxicity increase progressively as SDC exceed 20 μg/mL, while symptoms and signs of asthma are not effectively reduced at SDC below 10 μg/mL. In general the patient should be at steady-state (3–5 elimination half-lives) to ensure reliable interpretation of SDC results.

Estimated Time To Steady-State		
Adults	Non-smokers	~2d
	Smokers	1–2 d; increased in cardiac decomposition or hepatic failure
Children		1–2 d, depending on age
Infants		Half-life gradually decreases from newborn value to childhood level
Normal newborns		~5d
Neonates, premature		~6d

- Peak concentrations should be monitored periodically to ensure that they <u>do not</u> exceed the upper limit of the therapeutic range.

SAMPLE COLLECTION

Therapy	**When To Sample**
IV	♦ Prior to IV infusion (if patient has history of theophylline ingestion) ♦ 30 min after completion of loading dose to determine whether an additional loading dose is needed ♦ 4–6 h after beginning infusion ♦ 12–18 h after beginning infusion ♦ Repeat serum measurements as needed

Therapy	When To Sample
Chronic oral therapy	♦ Peak: Sampling time depends on preparation--2h after oral dose of solution or solid dosage form with rapid dissolution, 4h after a slow-release preparation, 3–7h after Theo-Dur dose Trough: Immediately before next oral dose

CLINICAL MONITORING PARAMETERS

- Auscultation of lung fields
- Heart rate and rhythm
- Pulmonary function
- Respiratory rate and rhythm

THERAPEUTICS

USUAL DOSING PARAMETERS

ACUTE IV THERAPY

All doses stated as aminophylline (80–85% theophylline)

PATIENT GROUP	INITIAL DOSE	DAILY MAINTENANCE	APPROXIMATE T½ NORMAL RENAL FUNCTION
Pediatric			
Children (> 9 yr; healthy)		0.55 mg/kg/h	
Children (1–9 yr)		1.0 mg/kg/h	
Infants (4–52 wk)		0.008 mg/kg/h x (age in wk)+0.2	
Neonatal Apnea	5 mg/kg	1.25 mg/kg q 12 h	Adjust subsequent dosage to achieve a peak concentration in the range of 5–10 μg/mL Steady-state may require 5–7 days of therapy
Adult			
Healthy nonsmokers	6 mg/kg IV over 30 min for all 3 groups	0.5 mg/kg/h	No prior theophylline in previous 24 h
Smokers		0.7 mg/kg/h	
Cardiac decompensation and/or liver dysfunction		0.25 mg/kg/h	
Healthy nonsmokers	3 mg/kg IV over 30 min for all 3 groups	0.5 mg/kg/h	Prior theophylline administration; obtain stat SDC and start IV infusion
Smokers		0.7 mg/kg/h	
Cardiac decompensation and/or liver dysfunction		0.25 mg/kg/h	

ORAL THERAPY
All doses stated as theophylline

PATIENT GROUP	INITIAL DOSE	DAILY MAINTENANCE	APPROXIMATE T½ NORMAL RENAL FUNCTION
Pediatric			
Neonates	1 mg/kg/12 h	3 mg/kg/d	
Premature			~30h
Normal newborn			~24h
Infants			
4–52 wk	8 mg/kg/d	Dose (mg/kg/ 24 h)=(0.3) x (age in wk) + 8.0	3–14 h
Children			
1–9 yr	16 mg/kg/d to 400 mg/d (whichever is less) for both age groups	24 mg/kg/d	Mean: 3.7 h (range: 2–10 h)
9–12 yr		20 mg/kg/d	4 h
Adolescents			
12–16 yr	16 mg/kg/d to 400 mg/d (whichever is less)	18 mg/kg/d to 900 mg/d (whichever is less)	~4-9 h
Adults			
Adults (>16 yr) Healthy, non-smoker	16 mg/kg/d to 400 mg/d (whichever is less) for all adult groups	13 mg/kg/d to 900 mg/d (whichever is less)	Mean: 8.7 h (range: 4–16 h)
Healthy, cigarette or marijuana smoker	same as above	13 mg/kg/d up to 900 mg/d (whichever is less)	4.4 h
Cardiac decompensation (including cor pulmonale) or liver failure	same as above	Dose not to exceed 400 mg/d before measuring SDC	20–30 h

CLINICAL COMMENTS

IV THERAPY

- Aminophylline = 85% anhydrous theophylline.
- Serum theophylline concentrations increase about 2 μg/mL for every 1 mg/kg increase in the loading dose initially (V_d ~0.5L/Kg).
- Theophylline exhibits dose-dependent elimination kinetics in some patients; as the metabolic pathways become saturated, a relatively small increase in dose can provoke a disproportionate rise in the SDC. Thus, any need for increases in SDC of the drug must be accomplished in small dosage increments, and further therapeutic drug monitoring is essential for all but small dosage changes, i.e., less than a 25% increase or decrease in dose.
- Ideally, the initial infusion will be started after the loading dose and SDC obtained at the beginning of the infusion and 4–8h later.
- Variability in the peak SDC resulting from a loading dose will occur to some degree because of the interpatient differences in the volume of distribution. Therefore, loading doses should be calculated to attain target SDC 10–15 μg/mL, the lower end of the therapeutic range, and administered slowly over 15–30 min to avoid transiently high blood levels before distribution into tissues occurs. During IV therapy, a blood sample is obtained 30 min after completion of the loading dose to determine whether an additional loading dose is needed.

ORAL DOSING

- Initiate intermittent oral therapy with a reliably absorbed, sustained-release theophylline formulation at a dose of about 16 mg/kg/d up to a maximum of 400 mg/d, whichever is less. (Dosage interval depends on absorption rate of theophylline preparation used and the patient's elimination characteristics.) For infants 4–52 wk old, start with 8 mg/kg/d using a liquid, alcohol-free formulation (e.g., Slo-Phyllin syrup).
- Increase dose, if tolerated, in 25% increments, at 3-day intervals, to a dose no higher than the limits shown on pages 91 and 92. Use ideal body weight for obese patients. If any adverse effects are present, then the next dose should be withheld and subsequent doses reduced.

♦ Slow-release theophylline preparations that are reliably and completely absorbed are the drugs of choice for chronic therapy. These commercially available preparations vary in their rate and completeness of absorption, however, and the dosing interval for these products should be based on both product absorption and patient elimination characteristics.

GENERAL

♦ Various theophylline formulations include theophylline as salts or as derivatives, therefore, the amount of anhydrous theophylline varies among different preparations. For example, aminophylline (theophylline ethylenediamine) contains from 78–86% theophylline and is the only salt form in which parenteral theophylline is available. Other theophylline salts such as oxtriphylline (Choledyl), theophylline calcium salicylate, and theophylline sodium glycinate have variable theophylline content and no specific therapeutic advantages and are not recommended. Theophylline is also available IV.

♦ Dyphylline (7–dihydroxypropyl theophylline) is a xanthine bronchodilator that does not dissociate into theophylline and has only about one-fifth the potency. (This compound is not detected by theophylline assays).

♦ Combinations of theophylline and phenobarbital should be avoided (see p. 129).

COMMON TOXICITIES AND ADVERSE REACTIONS

TOXICITY	INCIDENCE	CLINICAL COMMENTS
Serum Concentration 5–20 μg/mL		
Nausea, cramps, insomnia, headache	Rare	Duration transient if oral dose is slowly titrated over 1–2 wk
	Common, if therapeutic SDC are rapidly attained (loading dose)	Avoided by slow titration of dose when clinically feasible; duration transient
	Common, if ephedrine is concurrently administered	Avoid use of combination products, since ephedrine adds no benefit and toxicity is synergistic with theophylline; duration persistent
Tremors	Rare; occurs with concurrent administration of oral $beta_2$ agonists (e.g., terbutaline)	Avoided if the $beta_2$ agonist is inhaled rather than taken orally; duration unknown.
Excessive gastric acid secretion	Rare	May produce symptoms in a patient with an active gastric ulcer
Serum Concentration 15–35 μg/mL		
Nausea, vomiting, diarrhea, stomachache, headache, irritability, nervousness, insomnia, sinus tachycardia	Common, at SDC >20 μg/mL	Reduce dose immediately; duration persistent
Hyperglycemia	Rare	Duration persistent; may occur in neonates
Serum Concentration > 35 μg/mL		
Seizure, which may be intractable and unresponsive to anticonvulsants; cerebral hypoxia; cardiac arrhythmias; cardiorespiratory arrest; death	Common	Duration persistent; minor adverse effects (e.g., nausea) often do not precede life-threatening toxicity and cannot be relied upon as warning signs or dosing endpoint

DRUG INTERACTIONS

DRUG	MECHANISM	CLINICAL COMMENTS
Allopurinol	Possibly due to effect of allopurinol on liver microsomal enzymes	Modest ↑ in theophylline SDC possible
Antacids	Possible absorption of theophylline onto antacid or alteration of gastric emptying	↑ or ↓ in rate but not extent of absorption
Barbiturates	Induction of hepatic cytochrome microsomal enzyme system	↓ in serum theophylline concentration; it appears that administration of phenobarbital for several weeks is required for the interaction effect to become apparent
Cimetidine	↓ clearance	↑ in serum theophylline concentration; theophylline concentration may ↑ by 30–40% within the first 24 h; the slightly higher maximum effect is seen within 48–72 h
Ciprofloxacin	↓ clearance by competitive hepatic inhibition; ↑ T½ and SDC with toxicity has been observed in some patients	
Influenza A vaccine	Mechanism of possible effect is unknown	Possible ↑ in serum theophylline concentration
Isoproterenol	↓ serum theophylline level	Concomitant IV administration
Lithium	↑ excretion of lithium	↓ lithium level and possible decreased therapeutic effect
Macrolide antibiotics, troleandomycin, erythromycin salts and base	↓ of hepatic clearance peaking at 5–7 days after erythromycin is begun	↑ in serum theophylline concentration; generally not more than 25–35%
Oral contraceptives	Inhibits hepatic microsomal enzymes	↑ SDC; ↓ in theophylline clearance of approximately 30% has been reported in women taking oral contraceptives
Phenytoin	Induces cytochrome mixed-function oxidase activity	Patients with asthma and seizures requiring phenytoin therapy will require monitoring of serum theophylline concentration; adjust dosage to compensate for the accelerated metabolism of theophylline induced by phenytoin. Phenytoin concentration should also be measured. ↓ in theophylline SDC and ↓ in phenytoin SDC. Substantial ↑ in theophylline clearance (40–75%). After 10–14 days theophylline appears to ↓ rate of phenytoin absorption

DRUG	MECHANISM	CLINICAL COMMENTS
Propranolol	↓ theophylline clearance	Since asthmatic patients should usually not be treated with beta-blocking agents because of the potential for aggravation of the asthma, this observation is of limited clinical relevance. ↑ theophylline SDC, approximately 30%
Rifampin	Clearance ↑ after concurrent administration, probably due to hepatic induction	↓ theophylline SDC. ↑ clearance as much as 79%
Benzodiazepines, carbamazepine, diuretics, influenza vaccine, isoniazid, verapamil	Unknown	Isolated reports of possible alteration of serum theophylline concentration due to drug interaction has been reported with a number of other drugs. These reports require confirmation
$Beta_2$ agonists	Possible myocardial necrosis	The potential for an additive cardiovascular effect with theophylline-$beta_2$ agonist combination exists but has not been proven in humans
Ephedrine	Synergistic toxicity; mechanism is unknown	Increased symptoms of central nervous system excitation

CLINICAL INTERPRETATION

SDC data must be interpreted together with the patient's current clinical status, response, and pharmacokinetic considerations. A therapeutic level attained before steady-state may indicate a potentially toxic level when steady-state is reached.

Factors Decreasing Theophylline Concentrations

- Smoking (cigarettes or marijuana). Smokers have faster clearance than non-smokers.
- Children have faster clearance than non-smoking adults

Factors That May Increase Theophylline Serum Concentrations

- In neonates, plasma clearance rates are reduced; the half-life in infants gradually approaches normal childhood values over the first 8 months
- Cardiac decompensation (including cor pulmonale)
- Hepatic dysfunction
- Cessation of smoking (clearance gradually slows to non-smoking levels)
- Concomitant drug therapy: macrolide antibiotics, cimetidine, allopurinol (600 mg/d), or propranolol
- Fever associated with upper respiratory infection

VALPROIC ACID

CLINICAL PHARMACOKINETICS
SUMMARY TABLE

SERUM CONCENTRATIONS		
Minimum effective concentration		40–50 µg/mL
Potentially toxic concentration		>100 µg/mL
% BIOAVAILABILITY		90–100%
TIME TO PEAK CONCENTRATION	Syrup	0.5–1.0 h
	Capsules	1–3 h
	Enteric coated tablet	2–6 h (peak times are prolonged when administered with food)
TIME TO STEADY-STATE		1–3 d
HALF-LIFE (T½)	Adults	
	Comedication	6–12 h
	Monotherapy	8–20 h
	Liver disease	20–30 h
	Children	
	Comedication	3–12 h
	Monotherapy	7–14 h
VOLUME OF DISTRIBUTION		~0.2 L/kg (range: 0.1–0.5 L/kg)
CLEARANCE		
Total body clearance	Adults	
	Comedication	15 mL/h/kg
	Monotherapy	7–8 mL/h/kg
	Children	
	Comedication	25–30 mL/h/kg
	Monotherapy	15 mL/h/kg
% PROTEIN-BOUND		~90–95%
% EXCRETED RENALLY UNCHANGED		<5%
MAJOR ROUTE OF ELIMINATION	Hepatic	>90%
ACTIVE METABOLITES		Several unsaturated active metabolites; probably minor contribution to antiepileptic activity of valproic acid

THERAPEUTIC DRUG MONITORING

GENERAL GUIDELINES

- In general, determination of valproic acid SDC following the first dose are not indicated. Since valproic acid pharmacokinetics appear to be concentration-dependent, the most cost-efficient strategy involves achieving steady-state conditions before determining valproic acid concentrations. It is recommended that patients begin an initial dosage regimen and then have blood samples collected after 2–4 d of therapy.

- Wide variability and nonlinearity in valproic acid pharmacokinetics necessitate that dosage regimens be set according to the individual. Valproic acid SDC should be obtained 2–4 d after any change in valproic acid dosage or dosing interval. Indications for monitoring valproic acid SDC include the following: development of signs of toxicity, a decrease in seizure control, the addition or withdrawal of other antiepileptic drugs, or suspected non-compliance.

SAMPLE COLLECTION

SDC may fluctuate substantially during a dosing interval, necessitating multiple SDC determinations in some patients.

	WHEN TO SAMPLE	CLINICAL COMMENTS
Initial Monitoring		
♦ Following initiation of therapy	2–4 d after beginning treatment--peak or trough	Time to peak is delayed if taken immediately after meal
	~1.3h after dose, prior to next dose	Sampling both peak and trough SDC permits the clinician to adjust both the dosing interval and dose

	WHEN TO SAMPLE	CLINICAL COMMENTS
Resampling		
♦ Change in dose or dosing interval	2–4 d after change--peak and/or trough	Normal time to steady-state for adults: 30–85 h, for children: 20–70 h
♦ When other anti-epileptic drugs are added or withdrawn	Trough	
♦ Decrease in seizure control	Trough	
♦ Signs of toxicity	Peak	Laboratory or physical signs
♦ When non-compliance is suspected	Trough	

CLINICAL MONITORING PARAMETERS

- ♦ CBC with platelets
- ♦ Hepatic function at least every 2 months
- ♦ Renal function (periodically)

THERAPEUTICS

USUAL DOSING PARAMETERS

PATIENT GROUP	INITIAL DOSE	DAILY MAINTENANCE	APPROXIMATE T½ NORMAL RENAL FUNCTION
Pediatric			
Children			
Monotherapy	15 mg/kg/d	15–100 mg/kg (divided into 2–3 doses)	3–12 h
Comedication	15 mg/kg/d		7–20 h
Adults			
Monotherapy	5–10 mg/kg/d	15–45 mg/kg/d (as single or 2–3 divided doses)	8–20 h
Comedication	15 mg/kg/d		6–12 h

CLINICAL COMMENTS

- Oral valproic acid loading doses frequently cause significant gastroenteritis and are not tolerated by many patients.
- The dosing requirements for children tend to approach adult requirements at age 12.
- Patients with severe hepatic dysfunction require smaller doses and a different dosing frequency; half-life may be prolonged to 20–30 h in these patients. Patients taking other antiepileptic drugs may require larger doses than patients receiving valproic acid alone.
- 60 mg/kg/d is the FDA-approved maximum daily dosage; any adjustment to a dosage exceeding 60 mg/kg/d should be titrated with the aid of SDC.
- Enteric-coated preparation is not a sustained-release product; **however**, it does produce a lag phase and therefore a delay in the time to peak concentrations.
- Loading doses are not necessary under usual circumstances.
- Maintenance dose should be determined primarily on the response of each patient.

COMMON TOXICITIES AND ADVERSE REACTIONS

TOXICITY	INCIDENCE	CLINICAL COMMENTS
Dermatologic		
Hair loss	2–12%	Usually temporary; regrowth may be curly or altered in texture
Rash	Rare	Case report of macular pruritic rash
Gastrointestinal		
Anorexia	5%	
Nausea and vomiting	3%	With enteric-coated formulations incidence of nausea and vomiting is reduced
Pancreatitis	Rare	Asymptomatic elevation of amylase in 20% of children
Weight gain	8–18%	More common in adult females than males; may be as high as 44% in females
Hematologic		
Bone marrow suppression	Rare	Usually reversible (case report only)
Decreased fibrinogen	Rare	Usually reversible (case report only)
Neutropenia	Rare	Usually reversible (case report only)
Thrombocytopenia	6–40%	More common in children, dose-related, reversible

TOXICITY	INCIDENCE	CLINICAL COMMENTS
Hepatotoxicity		
Acute hepatotoxicity	Rare	More frequent in children with severe epilepsy, mental retardation, or brain damage (case report only)
Asymptomatic elevation of liver function tests	6–16%	Only 3% on monotherapy; may be as high as 44% in children
Metabolic		
Hyperammonemia	50%	Usually asymptomatic, but may cause confusion, stupor, and/or coma
Neurological		
Behavioral deterioration	2.4% in children 0.9% in adults	
Drowsiness	5–14% on multiple antiepileptic drugs 0.2–1.4% on monotherapy	
Paresthesias	1%	
Stupor, confusion, coma	Rare	May be secondary to elevated ammonia concentrations; case reports confounded by multiple antiepileptic drugs and increased phenobarbital concentrations
Tremor	0.5–12%	May be dose-related; fine to medium or benign essential

DRUG INTERACTIONS

DRUG	MECHANISM	CLINICAL COMMENTS
Carbamazepine Phenobarbital Phenytoin Primidone	Induction of liver enzymes	Induction of liver enzymes by other antiepileptic drugs results in increased valproic acid clearance. Dosage increase may be required depending on patient response.
Ethosuximide	Possible decrease in ethosuximide metabolism	Little effect seen in patients only on valproic acid and ethosuximide, while ethosuximide SDC may increase in patients on multiple antiepileptic drug therapy. SDC are reported to increase from 30–130%. Although significance of interaction remains to be determined, a decrease in the ethosuximide dose may be necessary.
Phenobarbital, primidone	Decrease in intrinsic clearance of phenobarbital	Addition of valproic acid to phenobarbital therapy frequently necessitates a 20–50% decrease in phenobarbital dose.
Phenytoin	(1) Valproic acid displaces phenytoin from a shared binding site on albumin, causing an increase in unbound phenytoin concentration (2) Valproic acid is capable of inhibiting phenytoin metabolism, causing an increase in unbound phenytoin concentration	These 2 mechanisms have opposing effects on total phenytoin concentrations and explain the observations of toxicity associated with "therapeutic" total concentrations.

CLINICAL INTERPRETATION

Factors Affecting Valproic Acid Serum Drug Concentrations

- Liver disease may increase SDC by decreasing Cl
- Discontinuation of concomitant antiepileptic drug therapy may increase SDC
- Age: children often have faster clearance than adults; may decrease SDC
- Concomitant drug therapy: phenytoin, phenobarbital, carbamazepine, or primidone; increases clearance (decreases SDC)
- Altered protein binding (hypoalbuminemia; decreased in uremia and liver disease): affects SDC-response relationship
- Complete response to therapy may be delayed up to 6 months after initiating therapy, despite optimal SDC; response to therapy affects SDC-response relationship

Other Keys to Interpretation

- SDC may fluctuate during a dosing interval, necessitating multiple SDC determinations in some patients
- Percent protein binding decreases as the valproic acid SDC increases
- Percent protein binding may be decreased in patients with uremia or liver disease
- Percent protein binding decreases in hypoalbuminemic states
- Peak: Generally 1–3 h after a dose (time to peak concentration is delayed if drug is taken immediately after meal)
- Valproic acid syrup is absorbed more rapidly than capsules
- Enteric-coated tablets have an absorption lag phase, making the time to peak concentration difficult to predict. Trough SDC are more informative

Normal Time to Steady-state

Adults	30–85 h
Children	20–70 h May be prolonged in patients with hepatic disease

VANCOMYCIN

CLINICAL PHARMACOKINETICS
SUMMARY TABLE

SERUM CONCENTRATIONS		
Minimum effective concentrations	Peak concentration	20–40 mcg/ml
	Trough concentration	2–12 mcg/ml
Potentially toxic concentrations	Peak concentration	>80 mcg/ml
	Trough concentration	>20 mcg/ml
TIME TO PEAK CONCENTRATION		~30-120 min after completion of infusion
TIME TO STEADY-STATE		20–30 h with chronic dosing
HALF-LIFE (T½)	Adults	4–10 h
	Pediatrics	
	Neonates	2–3 h
	Children	6–10 h
VOLUME OF DISTRIBUTION		
Adults		
Creatinine clearance		
<10 mL/min	1 compartment	0.5–1.4 L/kg
	2 compartment	0.2–0.6 L/kg
≥10–50 mL/min	1 compartment	0.6–1.9 L/kg
	2 compartment	0.3–1.3 L/kg
≥50–100 mL/min	1 compartment	0.4–1.4 L/kg
	2 compartment	0.2–1.4 L/kg
>100 mL/min	1 compartment	0.5–0.8 L/kg
	2 compartment	0.2–1.5 L/kg
Children	<1 wk old	~725mL/kg
	~3mo old	~650mL/kg
	~3yr old	~800mL/kg
	~5yr old	~750mL/kg
	~7yr old	~550mL/kg

		Vancomycin Clearance
CLEARANCE		
Total Body Clearance		
Adults		
<10 mL/min	1 compartment	1–16 mL/min
	2 compartment	13–33 mL/min
≥10–50 mL/min	1 compartment	6–63 mL/min
	2 compartment	25–95 mL/min
≥50–100 mL/min	1 compartment	15–104 mL/min
	2 compartment	43–110 mL/min
>100 mL/min	1 compartment	75–99 mL/min
	2 compartment	42–184 mL/min
Children (per 1.73 m^2)	3.3 d old	15 mL/min
	4.7 d old	27 mL/min
	2.6 mo old	30 mL/min
	3.1 mo old	50 mL/min
	≥3 yr old	163 mL/min
	≥5 yr old	131 mL/min
	≥7 yr old	134 mL/min
Dialysis Clearance		
Hemodialysis		Probably is clinically insignificant
Peritoneal dialysis		Requires dosage adjustment based on pre- and post-dialysis SDC
% PROTEIN-BOUND		~5%
% EXCRETED RENALLY UNCHANGED		80–90%
MAJOR ROUTE OF ELIMINATION	Renal	>90% unchanged in urine
ACTIVE METABOLITES		None known

THERAPEUTIC DRUG MONITORING

GENERAL GUIDELINES

- Use of vancomycin SDC and appropriate dosage adjustments are essential to optimize vancomycin therapy.

- The distribution phase (α-phase) of vancomycin complicates the serum sampling strategy. It is important that **consistency** be maintained in the dosage interval and infusion period throughout the course of vancomycin therapy.

- Peak serum samples must be performed uniformly at a pre-selected time post-infusion for subsequent comparisons to be valid. Comparing so-called peak concentrations drawn at 15 min post-infusion one day and 30 min post-infusion the next day is invalid. The slope of the SDC time curve during the distribution phase is very steep, and differences of as little as 15 min in sampling can result in 10–15 mg/L difference in measured vancomycin concentration.

- Variations in infusion period may also contribute to differences observed in measured vancomycin concentrations. The individual administering vancomycin must be directed to administer the drug using the same infusion period (including flushing the IV tube).

SAMPLE COLLECTION

- Generally, small samples of serum (≤50 μL) are required to perform quantitative vancomycin determination using contemporary assay techniques. Drawing of 1–2 mL of blood should provide the necessary volume of serum required for vancomycin analysis. The samples can be drawn in a standard red-top tube using a standard plastic syringe and needle. As with all drug samples, the serum should be separated then processed without delay after the blood has been drawn.

Therapy		**WHEN TO SAMPLE**
IV	Peak	30–120 min after the completion of a 60–min infusion
	Trough	Immediately prior to the next dose

CLINICAL MONITORING PARAMETERS

- Renal function S_{cr} and BUN
- Albumin
- CBC
- Auditory function prior to and during treatment

THERAPEUTICS

USUAL DOSING PARAMETERS

PATIENT GROUP	INITIAL DOSE	DAILY MAINTENANCE	APPROXIMATE T½ NORMAL RENAL FUNCTION
Pediatric			
Neonates	15 mg/kg	30 mg/kg/d (q 8–12 h)	4–10 h
Children	15–25 mg/kg	40–60 mg/kg/d (q 6–8 h)	2–3 h
Adult			
Normal renal function	25 mg/kg	20–40 mg/kg/d (q 6–8 h)	4–10 h
Impaired renal function	25 mg/kg	$15xC_{cr}+150$ mg/d (q 12–24 h)	1–3 d
Functionally anephric	15 mg/kg	15 mg/kg (q 7–10 d)	Prolonged > 3 d

CLINICAL COMMENTS

- ♦ Renal function will dictate daily maintenance.
- ♦ Hemodialysis does not significantly affect maintenance dose recommendations.
- ♦ Peritoneal dialysis requires a variable adjustment and should be guided by pre- and post-dialysis monitoring for each patient.
- ♦ Vancomycin should be added to D_5W or 0.9% NaCl solutions and infused IV over 60 min.

COMMON TOXICITIES AND ADVERSE REACTIONS

TOXICITY	INCIDENCE	CLINICAL COMMENTS
Nephrotoxicity		
with amino-glycoside	35%	Usually reversible Patients with poor renal function may develop nephrotoxicity rapidly
without amino-glycoside	5%	
Neutropenia	2%	
Ototoxicity	<1%	Age and/or renal function may be risk factors; definition for auditory toxicity poorly defined in many of the early studies
Phlebitis	13%	Fairly common--should try administering vancomycin with a large diluent volume over at least 1 h
Rash	3%	Macular papular
Red-neck syndrome	35% in children	Pseudoanaphylactoid infusion-related reaction, usually begins 10 min after infusion and resolves in 15–20 min

DRUG INTERACTIONS

DRUG	MECHANISM	CLINICAL COMMENTS
Aminoglycosides Amphotericin B Cephalosporins Cisplatin Cyclosporine Ethacrynic acid Furosemide	Additive ototoxicity and/or nephrotoxicity may occur with each of these agents	May be reversible. Serial audiometric determinations may be required. Monitor renal function closely.

CLINICAL INTERPRETATION

- ♦ SDC-time data must be interpreted together with the patient's current clinical status, response, and pharmacokinetic considerations.

- ♦ Renal disease may increase SDC.

- ♦ Due to the pronounced bi-exponential decay of the vancomycin SDC time curve, this drug does not lend itself to the traditional pharmacokinetic approaches. Vancomycin may require multiple samplings during both the distribution and elimination curves. However, most clinicians obtain SDC only during elimination phases.

- ♦ The distribution phase (α-phase) of vancomycin complicates the serum sampling strategy. It is important that **consistency** be maintained in the dosage interval and infusion period throughout the course of vancomycin therapy.

- ♦ Peak serum samples must be performed uniformly at a pre-selected time post-infusion for subsequent comparisons to be valid. <u>Comparing so-called peak concentrations drawn at 15 min post-infusion one day and 30 min post-infusion the next day is invalid.</u> The slope of the SDC time curve during the distribution phase is very steep, and differences of as little as 15 min in sampling can result in 10–15 mg/L difference in measured vancomycin concentration.

- ♦ In situations where the patient is receiving vancomycin every 6h, 30–60 min of the dosage interval is utilized for infusion of the drug, 2–3h of the dosage interval are required in order to complete distribution, leaving only 2–3h to characterize the terminal portion of the SDC time curve. Optimizing the characterization of the terminal half-life may require extending serum sampling through approximately 1.5 terminal half-lives and withholding a dose of vancomycin in patients with suspected or documented sepsis. The alternative is trying to characterize half-life using 2–3h of SDC time data at a point at which the average patient has a terminal drug half-life of 6h.

- ♦ Blood urea nitrogen and serum creatinine samples should be obtained weekly during vancomycin therapy.

- ♦ Audiometric testing should be considered for patients who are suspected to be at high risk of vancomycin ototoxicity.

- ♦ Special precautions should be taken to use relatively dilute solutions of vancomycin and to infuse the drug over 60 min.

- ♦ Careful attention should be given to rotating peripheral IV sites to minimize the possibility of phlebitis.

PHARMACOKINETIC TABLES

RATES OF ELIMINATION

DRUG	MAJOR ROUTE OF ELIMINATION
Amikacin	Renal
Carbamazepine	Hepatic
Digoxin	Renal
Digitoxin	Hepatic
Gentamicin	Renal
Tobramycin	Renal
Lidocaine	Hepatic
Lithium	Renal
Phenobarbital	Hepatic
Primidone	Hepatic
Phenytoin	Hepatic
Procainamide	Renal excretion Hepatic metabolism
Quinidine	Hepatic
Theophylline	Renal excretion Hepatic
Valproic Acid	Hepatic
Vancomycin	Renal

DIALYSIS OF DRUGS

DRUG	HEMO-DIALYSIS	PERITONEAL DIALYSIS	HEMO-PERFUSION	COMMENTS
Amikacin	D (50-100%)	ND (0-5%)	N/A	50-70% of the LD may be given post-dialysis
Carbamazepine	N/A	N/A	D (20-50%)	
Digoxin	ND	ND	D	
Digitoxin	ND	ND		
Gentamicin	D (50-100%)	ND (0-5%)	N/A	50-70% of the LD may be given post-dialysis
Tobramycin	D (50-100%)	ND	N/A	50-70% of the LD may be given post-dialysis
Lidocaine	ND	N/A	N/A	
Lithium	D	D	N/A	
Phenobarbital	D (30%)	D	D	Usual dose post-HD
Primidone	D (30%)	N/A	N/A	
Phenytoin	ND	ND	D	
Procainamide	D			
Quinidine	D	D		
Theophylline	N/A	N/A	D	
Valproic Acid	ND	ND		
Vancomycin	ND	D	D	

D = Dialyzed
N/A = Not Available
ND = Not Dialyzed

CONSIDERATIONS WHEN SELECTING A PHARMACOKINETICS SOFTWARE PROGRAM

VENDOR

- Reputation of Software Vendor
- Professional and Technical Personnel on Staff
- Quality Verified through Published Clinical Research
- Years of Service
- Number of Installations
- Mission of Software Vendor
- Hardware Requirements
- Operating Platform
- License/Maintenance Fees

SUPPORT

- On-line Help Embedded within Software
- Clinical Consultant Service Availability
- Technical Consultant Service Availability
- Software Fully Error Trapped with Escape Key/Back Up
- Update Availability and Frequency
- Responsiveness to User Enhancement Suggestions
- Software Training Materials/Service Availability
- Pharmacokinetics/TDM Training Availability
- Case Studies Available with Professional Feedback
- Ease of Training/Use
- Quality of Reference and Training Manuals
- References/Descriptions of All Equations Utilized
- References/Descriptions of All Age, Drug, Disease, Habit Effects

KINETIC MODELS

- Kinetic Parameter Limitations/Warnings
- Comprehensiveness as to Age, Interactions, Dosage Forms
- User Selectable Model/Modify Parameters
- Generic Model Availability
- Number of Drugs Available
- Drugs Available that meet Site Requirements
- Flexibility in Simulating Clinical Realities
- Adjustments for Changing Renal Function
- Adjustments for Interactions Stopped/Started
- Flexibility in Curve Fitting Approaches (linear, non-linear, Bayesian, Michaelis-Menten)

REPORTS

- Patient Data Storage
- Database Management
- Customized Reports as to Text and Format
- Ability to Save, Reuse, Modify Standard Text for Reports
- Graphics
- Drug Monographs
- Managerial Statistics
- Prescribing Feedback Programs
- Ability to Evaluate Impact of Interaction on Quality of Care

SYSTEM INTERNATIONAL CONVERSION CHART

UNITS CONVERSION CHART

The conversion from µg/mL to µmoles/L (International Units) is done using the following formula:

$$\text{Drug concentration } (\mu g/mL) \times \frac{1000}{\text{Molecular weight of the drug (g/mole)}} = \mu moles/L$$

Drug (Molecular Weight)	Recommended Serum Drug Concentrations* µg/mL	µmol/L
Amikacin (1.72)	20–30 (peak) 1–4 (trough)	34.7–53.8 1.7–7.2
Carbamazepine (236.26)	4.0–8.0 (multiple drug regimen) 8.0–12.0 (single drug)	17–34 34.51
Digoxin (780.92)	0.08–2.0 ng/mL	1.2–2.6 nmol/L
Gentamicin/ Tobramycin ****	0.1–2 (trough) 5–12 (peak)	
Lidocaine (234.33)	1.5–5.0	6.2
Lithium (6.94)	0.3–1.3 mEq/L	0.3–1.3 mmol/L
Phenobarbital (232.23)	15.0–40.0	65–172
Phenytoin (252.26)	10.0–20.0** (Adults & Children)	40–80
Primidone (218.25)	5.0–12.0	23–55

Drug (Molecular Weight)	Recommended Serum Drug Concentrations* µg/mL	µmol/L
Procainamide (271.79)	4.0–10.0	15–37
Quinidine (324.41)	2.3–5.0***	7–15***
Theophylline (180.17)	10.0–20.0 (asthma) 5.0–10.0 (apnea)	55–111 28–55
Valproic Acid (144.21)	50–100	347–693
Vancomycin ****	2–12 (trough) 20–40 (peak)	1.4–8.3 13.8–27.6

* The concentrations stated in this table are intended for interpretation of international literature and offer a general guide to the desirable SDC. Please see individual drugs for specific information.

** 6–14 µg/mL (24–55 µmol/L) for pre-term neonates and infants to 12 weeks.

*** Varies with assay method. Listed range is for double extraction fluorometric method.

**** No known molecular weight

GLOSSARY

GLOSSARY

Absorption: The process by which a drug enters the body. Intravascularly administered drugs are absorbed totally, but extravascular administration yields varying degrees and rates of absorption. The rate of absorption is calculated using the SDC-versus-time curve. Drugs are usually absorbed by passive diffusion of the nonionized drug fraction. The relationship between the rate of absorption and the rate of elimination is the principal determinant of the drug concentration in the bloodstream.

Accumulation: Repetitive dosing at timed intervals (before the previously administered dose has been completely cleared) causes a gradual increase in the SDC until steady-state is reached. The extent of accumulation is a function of the ratio of the dosage interval and the drug's half-life. Drug accumulation continues until the amount of drug eliminated per dosage interval equals the amount administered during that time.

Bioavailability: The portion of the drug dose that is available to enter the systemic circulation.

Clearance: The removal of a drug or endogenous substrate from a biologic system, such as serum and/or tissue. Clearance represents the hypothetical volume of distribution that is cleared in a given time period and is usually expressed as milliliters per minute (mL/min) or liters per hour (L/h). In kinetic terms, body clearance is the product of the volume of distribution and the elimination rate constant, which is the slope of the natural logarithm of the SDC-versus-time curve.

Compartment: A mathematical concept used to describe the distribution characteristics of a given drug in the body. A one-compartment model suggests immediate equilibrium between the serum and tissue concentrations of a drug. In reality, however, two or more compartments may be necessary to suggest the time required to achieve equilibrium within various body fluids, organs, and tissues. Occasionally, more complicated multi-compartment models must be used to describe a drug's elimination characteristics.

Creatinine Clearance (C_{cr}): The ratio of the rate of creatinine excretion in urine to its concentration in the serum. Decreased creatinine clearance, which occurs in renal dysfunction and with advancing age, must be considered when administering drugs that are cleared by the kidneys.

$$C_{cr} \text{ for males} = \frac{\text{weight in kg x (140 - patient's age)}}{\text{72 x serum creatinine}}$$

$$C_{cr} \text{ for females} = \frac{\text{0.85 x weight in kg x (140 - patient's age)}}{\text{72 x serum creatinine}}$$

Dialysis: The clearance of drug by a hemodialysis unit. The magnitude of dialysis is highest for water-soluble drugs that are not highly bound to serum proteins. For dialysis to significantly remove a large fraction of drug from the body within a reasonable period of time, dialysis must make a significant contribution to body clearance, and the drug must have a relatively small volume of distribution.

Disposition: The sum of distribution and elimination, which comprises both the alpha and beta portions of the declining SDC-versus-time curve. Disposition thus details the post-absorptive "fate" of an agent.

Distribution: The dispersion of the systemically available drug from the intravascular space into extravascular fluids and tissues and thus to the target receptor site. The process is represented on the SDC-versus-time curve by the alpha phase or early portion of the declining curve.

Dose Dependence: The change in certain pharmacokinetic parameters (that are usually constant) as a function of administered dose or SDC. Also known as concentration dependence. The physiological processes that influence dose-dependent parameters are generally capacity-limited. Clearance, elimination half-life, and bioavailable fraction are parameters that may be dose- or concentration-dependent. See also **Michaelis-Menten Kinetics** and **Zero-Order Kinetics**.

Dose Rate: A term indicating the amount of drug administered per unit time, without regard to frequency of intermittent dosing. Dose rate may be expressed as a daily dose (mg/d), or in smaller units of time (mg/min or mg/h). The dose rate of 1.44 grams per day may be administered as a constant infusion (i.e., 1 mg/min) or it may be given intermittently (i.e., 180 mg every 3h or 360 mg every 6h). The dose rate needed to achieve a desired average steady-state concentration is chosen based on knowledge of the bioavailable fraction and body clearance of the drug.

Dose-Response Curve: A graphic representation of the effectiveness or toxicity of a drug (i.e., response) versus the dose administered. The curve is sigmoid (S-shaped), with a straight line midsection, where there exists a log relationship with drug dose and effect. The lower part of the sigmoid curve represents a subtherapeutic SDC while the upper part represents a plateau effect with no ↑ effect of drug, but possible toxicity.

Dosing Interval: The frequency of intermittent drug administration. Once a dose rate is chosen, the appropriate dosing interval is chosen based on the half-life of the drug. Shorter dosing intervals (more frequent administration) are generally chosen for drugs with short elimination half-lives, while once-daily doses may be sufficient for drugs with long elimination half-lives. Short half-life drugs that are formulated with prolonged-release characteristics may also be given at longer dosing intervals. The appropriate dose to be administered at each dosing interval is determined by the product of dose rate and dosing interval.

Elimination Rate Constant: The fraction of the volume of distribution that may be cleared per unit of time. The elimination rate constant (K_{el}) is determined by dividing 0.693 by the half-life (T½): $K_{el} = 0.693/T½$. The sum of all the processes that terminate the presence of a drug in the body. The principal routes of drug elimination from the body are through the kidneys (glomerular filtration and tubular secretion) and the liver (biotransformation). Elimination through the biliary tract, the lungs, and sweat glands also occurs.

Enterohepatic Recirculation (Biliary Recycling): Drugs and metabolites that are excreted through bile into the intestine may be reabsorbed from the intestinal lumen into the portal circulation and thus re-enter the bloodstream.

Enzyme Induction: An increase in microsomal enzyme content or the rate of enzymatic processes, which results in more rapid metabolism of a compound. Certain drugs (e.g., phenytoin) may stimulate enzyme production. Drug clearance may be increased and the biologic half-life decreased.

Enzyme Inhibition: A decrease in the rate of metabolism of a compound through inhibition of metabolic enzyme systems. Inhibition may be caused by drugs competing for the same enzyme system or by specific inhibitors such as isoniazid, chloramphenicol, and dicumarol. Half-life may be increased and drug clearance decreased.

Excretion: The final elimination of an agent from the body's systemic circulation through the kidney into urine, bile into feces, saliva, and sweat.

First-Order Kinetics: The transfer of a constant fraction or percentage of a drug per unit time. Such passive functions as absorption and glomerular filtration proceed by first-order kinetics. In first-order kinetics, the quantity being processed is directly proportional to the amount of drug that remains to be processed. (See also **Zero-Order Kinetics**.) The following decline of the SDC of a drug with a 6h half-life illustrates a first-order process: The initial concentration of 40 μg/mL falls to 20 μg/mL at 6h, to 10 μg/mL at 12h, and to 5 μg/mL at 18h.

First-Pass Effect or Metabolism: The removal of a fraction of drug dose by the liver before it reaches the systemic circulation. The bioavailable fraction of a drug that undergoes first-pass metabolism is less than one and is lowest for drugs with high hepatic extraction ratios such as propranolol or nitroglycerin. Only drugs that are cleared by the liver and are administered by first-pass routes such as oral and rectal will undergo first-pass metabolism. These routes are uniquely first-pass because blood draining the sites of administration (i.e., gut and deep rectum) passes through the liver before reaching the general circulation. Drugs administered by routes that are not first-pass will have bioavailable fractions that are equal to one (i.e., intravenous route), or that are determined solely by the extent of absorption (i.e., sublingual or transdermal routes).

Free Drug Concentration: See **Unbound Drug Concentration.**

Half-Life: The time required for the SDC to decline by 50%.

$$\text{Half-life} = \frac{0.693 \times \text{volume of distribution}}{\text{clearance}}$$

Hepatic Clearance: The hypothetical calculation of the volume of distribution (in liters) of unmetabolized drug cleared through the liver in one minute (L/min).

Hepatic Metabolism: Most drugs are subject to chemical alterations by the body. The greatest number of these chemical reactions occur in the liver; reactions also occur in many other tissues and organs. Microsomal enzyme systems located in the liver catalyze glucuronide conjugations and drug oxidations, as well as drug reduction and hydrolysis.

International Units:
(See Conversion Chart)

$$\frac{\text{drug concentration } (\mu g/mL) \times 10^3}{\text{molecular wt of drug } (g/mole)}$$

LADME: An acronym that denotes various processes that influence SDC following drug administration (Liberation, Absorption, Distribution, Metabolism, and Excretion).

Lean Body Weight: The body weight of a patient minus the fat. Organ and body clearances are generally more closely related to lean body weight than total body weight and may be expressed as clearance per unit of lean body weight. Volumes of distribution for drugs that penetrate poorly into fatty tissue are better related to lean body weight than to total body weight and may be expressed as volume per unit of lean body weight. Lean body weight can be estimated by measuring height, weight, and girth of a patient. Ideal body weight is more commonly used for normalization of clearances or volumes and can be estimated by various formulas that take into consideration the height and sex of a patient.

Liberation: The release and dissolution of drug from its dosage form.

Loading Dose: The dose used initially to provide rapid therapeutic concentrations by eliminating the time required to achieve a steady-state with maintenance doses. The advisability of administering a loading dose should be determined based upon the drug's biologic half-life, dosing interval, the therapeutic concentrations to be achieved, and the clinical status of the patient. Monitor for therapeutic response as well as adverse drug reactions.

Maintenance Dose: A dosage regimen designed for chronic therapy. See also **Dose Rate** and **Dosing Interval.**

Metabolism: The chemical conversion or biotransfer of drugs or endogenous compounds into their respective metabolites by Phase I reactions (i.e., oxidation, reduction, hydrolysis) or Phase II synthetic reactions (i.e., acetylation, sulfation, glucuronidation). Most metabolism of drugs takes place in the liver through the action of hepatic microsomal enzyme systems. Because there is a limited number of enzymes in the liver available to interact with a drug, metabolism is a capacity-limited process and is capable of approaching a saturation limit. Hepatic clearance in this situation decreases with increasing dose rate or SDC and is characterized by Michaelis-Menten Kinetics.

Michaelis-Menten Kinetics: A set of equations that describes the rate of drug metabolism by a capacity-limited or saturable process as a function of 2 constants (V_{max} and K_m) and 1 variable (drug concentration). The Michaelis constant, K_m, is the concentration of drug at which the rate of metabolism is half maximal; V_{max} is the maximum rate of metabolism and is based on the number of metabolizing enzymes. Drugs that are characterized by Michaelis-Menten Kinetics (e.g., phenytoin) show disproportionate increases in average steady-state drug concentrations with increase in dose rate and must be carefully monitored.

Minimum Effective Concentration: The minimum SDC necessary to produce a desired pharmacologic effect in the majority of patients. Also, the lowest value of the therapeutic range. Although a therapeutic response may be seen at this level, the actual point at which patients respond is highly individual. Many patients may require titration to a higher level within the therapeutic range to obtain a beneficial pharmacologic response.

Nonlinear Kinetics: See also **Dose Dependence** and **Zero-Order Kinetics.**

Peak Serum Concentration (C_{max}): The point of maximum concentration on the SDC-versus-time curve.

Pharmacokinetics. The quantitative study of the metabolic processes and relationships between a drug dose and drug concentration in biologic fluids.

Potentially Toxic Concentrations: SDC associated with the onset of dose-related toxicities. Because some patients require levels in the upper portion of the therapeutic range for optimal therapy, caution is warranted whenever the SDC nears the upper boundary of the therapeutic range with drugs where the appearance of side effects closely correlates with SDC.

Protein Binding: The phenomenon that occurs when a drug combines with plasma or tissue protein to form a reversible complex. Protein binding is a dynamic process and depends on the drug's affinity for the protein molecule, the concentrations of protein and drug, and the number of protein binding sites. Drugs can be displaced from binding sites by other compounds that have a higher affinity for those sites.

Renal Clearance: The hypothetical calculation of plasma volume in liters of unmetabolized drug cleared through the kidney per unit of time. Renal blood flow, urinary pH, and tubular resorption and secretion may all affect renal clearance.

Serum Concentration: The concentration of a substance that appears in the bloodstream. Routine measurements of SDC represent the sum of the free or unbound portion, which is believed to be the pharmacologically active fraction, and the protein-bound fraction.

Serum Concentration-Versus-Time Profile: A plot of serum drug (or metabolite) concentration (Y-axis) against time (X-axis) following a single dose or during a dosing interval. The shape of the curve depends on the rate of drug input by absorption or infusion and the rate of elimination.

The area under the curve depends on the administered dose, the bioavailable fraction, and body clearance.

Steady-State Serum Concentration (C_{ss}): Those values that recur with each dose once equilibrium is achieved between the amount of drug administered and the amount eliminated within a given time interval. For most drugs, a clinically significant steady-state is achieved after 3–5 elimination half-lives.

Steady-State Volume of Distribution: The only volume of distribution that is characterized by true physiologic volumes (blood volume or vascular space and tissue volume or extravascular space) and the relative binding of drug to proteins in these spaces. The steady-state volume of distribution can be calculated from SDC-versus-time data. With knowledge of the unbound drug fraction in serum and the steady-state volume, the fraction of drug in the body that is extravascular can be estimated.

Therapeutic Range: The range of the concentrations associated with a high degree of efficacy and a low risk of dose-related toxicity. Therapeutic range is a statistical concept; it is the concentration range associated with therapeutic response while maintaining a minimal risk of toxicity in a majority of patients.

Total Body Clearance: The rate of drug removal from the body, considered as a single unit. Total body clearance, which is the sum of renal clearance and metabolic clearance, becomes clinically relevant when the primary route of elimination is impaired. The value is usually expressed as units of volume per unit time.

Total Drug Concentration: The sum of the concentrations of free drug and protein-bound drug in plasma or serum.

Trapezoidal Rule: A mathematical formula used to calculate the area under a SDC-versus-time curve by dividing the curve into individual trapezoids (rectangles) and summing the areas of all. Each trapezoid area is determined as the product of the time interval between two serial samples and the mean of the corresponding SDC.

Trough Serum Concentration (C_{min}): The minimum concentration of the drug on the SDC-versus-time curve. Trough concentrations are theoretically present in the period immediately preceding administration of the next dose.

Unbound Drug: The fraction of drug in serum that is not bound to proteins. The unbound or "free" drug is believed to be the pharmacologically active portion that exerts the pharmacologic effect at the receptor site. The equilibrium between unbound and bound drug is reversible; thus the unbound, pharmacologically active fraction may increase while the SDC remains constant or falls (e.g., because of competition between drugs for the same binding site).

Volume of Distribution (V_d): A hypothetical volume of body fluid that would be required to dissolve the total amount of drug needed to achieve the same concentration as that found in the blood. Volume of distribution is thus a proportionality constant that relates the amount of drug in the body to that in the serum.

Zero-Order Kinetics: A process that occurs at a constant rate, independent of concentration. Constant-rate infusions are referred to as zero-order infusions. The liberation of drug from some sustained release oral dosage forms occurs as a zero-order process.

REFERENCES AND SUGGESTED READINGS

REFERENCES AND SUGGESTED READINGS

1. Robinson JD, Charache P. Introduction to Therapeutic Drug Monitoring and Pharmacokinetics. In: Taylor WJ, Diers Caviness MH, eds. A Textbook for the Clinical Application of Therapeutic Drug Monitoring. Irving, TX: Abbott Laboratories, Diagnostics Division. 1986:2.

2. Robinson JD, Lopez LM, Stewart WL. How to establish a pharmacokinetic consulting service for ambulatory patients. *Am J Hosp Pharm*. 1984;41:2048-56.

3. Robinson JD, Hatton RC, Russell WL, Klapp D, Lopez LM. Accuracy of serum gentamicin concentration predictions generated by a personal-computer software system. *Clin Pharm*. 1984;3:509.

4. Robinson JD Taylor WJ. Interpretation of Serum Drug Concentrations. In: Taylor WJ, Diers Caviness MH, eds. A Textbook for the Clinical Application of Therapeutic Drug Monitoring. Irving, TX: Abbott Laboratories, Diagnostics Division. 1986;31-45.

5. Taylor WJ, Finn AL, eds. Individualizing drug therapy: Practical applications of drug monitoring. Vol. 1. New York, NY: Gross, Townsend, Frank, Inc. 1981.

6. Evans WE, Oellerich M. Therapeutic drug monitoring clinical guide. Irving, TX: Abbott Laboratories. 1984.

7. Taylor WJ, Finn AL, Gotcher S. Individualizing drug therapy: Clinical notes on the application of drug monitoring. New York, NY: Gross, Townsend, Frank, Inc. 1981.

8. Rich DS Jeffrey LP. Pharmacokinetic consultation services: 1979 versus 1983. *Am J Hosp Pharm*. 1984:41-56. Letter.

9. Taylor JT, McLean AJ, Leonard RG, et al. Initial experience of clinical pharmacology and clinical pharmacy interactions in a clinical pharmacokinetics consultation service. *J Clin Pharmacol*. 1979;19:1-7.

10. Gibaldi M. Biopharmaceutics and Clinical Pharmacokinetics. Philadelphia, PA: Lean and Febiger. 1984.

11. Evans WE, Schentag JJ, Jusko WJ. Applied Pharmacokinetics: Principles of Therapeutic Drug Monitoring. Vancouver, WA: Applied Therapeutics, Inc. 1987.

12. Gehlbach SH, Wilkinson WE, Hammond WE, et al. Improving drug prescribing in a primary care practice. *Med Care*. 1984;22:192-201.

13. Svirbely JR, Speicher CE. The importance of requests and report forms in the interpretation of therapeutic drug monitoring. *Ther Drug Monit*. 1980;2:211-4.

14. Finn AL, Taylor WJ, Kane WJ. General principles: Practical applications of serum concentration monitoring. In: Taylor WJ, Finn AL, eds. Individualizing drug therapy: Practical applications of drug monitoring. New York, NY: Gross, Townsend, Frank, Inc. 1981:1-30.

15. Finn AL, Taylor WJ, Moore AL. Pharmaco-therapeutics for the family physician. *Am Fam Physician*. 1979;7:1-48.

16. Sawchuk RJ, Zaske DE, Cipolle RJ, et al. Kinetic model for gentamicin dosing with the use of individual patient parameters. *Clin Pharmacol Ther*. 1977;21:362.

17. Mungall D, Marshall J, Penn D, et al. Individualizing theophylline therapy: The impact of clinical pharmacokinetics on patient outcomes. *Ther Drug Monit*. 1983;5:95-113.

18. Taylor WJ. Pharmacokinetics. *Am J Med Tech*. 1983;49:557-63.

19. Rietscha WJ, Heissler JF, Paulson JF, Stockman RA, Bessert JA, Melby MJ. Collaborative clinical pharmacokinetics service in a community hospital. *Am J Hosp Pharm*. 1984;41:473-7.

20. Stargel WW, Roe CR, Routledge PA, Shand DG. Importance of blood collection tubes in plasma lidocaine determinations. *Clin Chem*. 1979;25:617-9.

21. Taylor WJ, Diers Caviness MH, eds. A Textbook for the Clinical Application of Therapeutic Drug Monitoring. Irving, TX: Abbott Laboratories, Diagnostics Division. 1986.

22. Svirbely JR, Speicher CE. The importance of request report forms in the interpretation of therapeutic drug monitoring. *Ther Drug Monit*. 1980;2:221-4.

23. Speicher CE, Smith JW. Interpretive reporting in clinical pathology. *JAMA*. 1980;243:1556-60.

24. Robinson JD. Pharmacokinetic services for ambulatory patients. *Am J Hosp Pharm*. 1981;38:1713-6.

25. Biller JA, Yeager AM, eds. The Harriet Lane Handbook. The Harriet Lane Service, Children's Medical and Surgical Center, Johns Hopkins Hospital, Ninth Edition, Year Book Medical Publishers, Inc., 1981.